And that they may **RECOVER** themselves out of the snare
of the devil, who are taken captive by him at his will.

- 2 Timothy 2:26

A Doctor's Discovery & Records of Recovery

ADDICTION

THE FACTS

Dr. George T. Crabb, D.O.
Steven B. Curington

A special thanks to the RU editorial team for tirelessly working to produce this product with us: Donna Bowman, Carolyn Curington, Joy Kingsbury, Kay Niederwerfer, Wendy Burks.

Design and Layout: Jeremy N. Jones, Benjamin A. Smith

REFORMERS UNANIMOUS RECOVERY MINISTRIES

PO Box 15732, Rockford, IL 61132
Visit our website at www.reformersrecovery.org
Printed in Canada

Crabb, Dr. George T., 1965-
Curington, Steven B., 1965-2010

Addiction - The Facts
ISBN 978-0-9761498-3-5

TABLE OF CONTENTS

INTRODUCTION
RU Addicted?

Addiction: medically speaking from a biblical perspective

The enormous question that faces us today is this: "Is addiction a disease?" The answer is: NO! Addiction is not a disease. But, it is a disorder. It is a disorder that can make you very sick both physically and spiritually. It is also the reason why many contract diseases. The disorder of addiction is brought on by a bad choice that is followed by many other bad choices.

I like to formally define addiction as "something I continue to do, even though I know it is bad for me." My friend, if you know it is bad for you, and you continue to do it, then you have a full fledged addiction. This disorder caused by addiction is a self-induced disorder of the brain. It is brought on when an individual improperly uses chemical substances and/or destructive behaviors as coping mechanisms to deal with the pain, uncertainty, disappointments, loss, and other like traumas in life.

As this behavior is repeated, physiological changes eventually occur in the brain. These changes further enhance the disorder and compel the individual to use the substance and/or destructive behavior with greater frequency and intensity. Eventually, the behavior leads to more pain, frustration, fear, uncertainty, and disappointment. The individual becomes trapped in a vicious cycle with unresolved pain as a result of engaging destructive coping mechanisms that were initially meant to alleviate the pain.

Addiction is a process that starts with a choice. That choice allows the manipulation of neurotransmitters (chemical messengers in the brain). However, through manipulation of these "feel goods," they are eventually depleted. This results in devastating destruction, depression, and ultimately death. Thus, the chasing of the "high" ends up being a futile struggle to maintain normality.

Addiction often finds its origin in a sense of personal dissatisfaction. Disappointment, anger, resentment, low self-esteem, rejection, and a host of other negative perceptions can lead an individual to search for redemption and relief in drugs, alcohol, and other self-destructive behaviors. At first, the individual discovers that the chemical or behavior not only offers relief from negative feelings, but it also offers a temporary sense of control and power.

Once the destructive behavior becomes a habit, however, the user quickly loses control and becomes the victim. Physically and emotionally dependent as well as spiritually bankrupt, the individual becomes virtually enslaved to the substance or behavior.

Because of the spiritual and emotional root causes of substance abuse and destructive behavior, along with the physical sequelae, the path to recovery must involve both spiritual, emotional, and physical correction and healing.

A life broken by substance abuse can be rebuilt, and an individual can emerge a stronger person. But, it is going to take the Truth! This book seeks to explain to you to the medical truth of your addiction, while at the same time introducing you to the spiritual Truth which will strengthen you out of your world of despair.

It is our wish that the Truth will make you free, that you may be FREED INDEED!

WHAT DOES THE BIBLE SAY
ABOUT ADDICTION?

"Know ye not, that to whom ye yield yourselves servants to obey, his servants ye are to whom ye obey; whether of sin unto death, or of obedience unto righteousness?"

Romans 6:16

"Knowing this, that our old man is crucified with him, that the body of sin might be destroyed that henceforth we should not serve sin."

Romans 6:6-7

"Then said Jesus to those Jews which believed on him, If ye continue in my word, then are ye my disciples indeed; And ye shall know the truth, and the truth shall make you free. They answered him, we be Abraham's seed, and were never in bondage to any man: how sayest thou, Ye shall be made free? Jesus answered them, Verily, verily, I say unto you, Whosoever committeth sin is the servant of sin."

John 8:31-34

"And he said unto me, My grace is sufficient for thee: for my strength is made perfect in weakness. Most gladly therefore will I rather glory in my infirmities, that the power of Christ may rest upon me."

2 Corinthians 12:9

"If the Son therefore shall make you free, ye shall be free indeed."

John 8:36

"For we know that the law is spiritual: but I am carnal, sold under sin For that which I do I allow not: for what I would, that do I not; but what I hate, that do I. If then I do that which I would not, I consent unto the law that it is good. Now then it is no more I that do it, but sin that dwelleth in me. For I know that in me (that is, in my flesh,) dwelleth no good thing: for to will is present with me; but how to perform that which is good I find not. For the good that I would I do not: but the evil which I would not, that I do. Now if I do that I would not, it is no more I that do it, but sin that dwelleth in me. I find then a law, that, when I would do good, evil is present with me."

Romans 7:14-21

"Know ye not that the unrighteous shall not inherit the kingdom of God? Be not deceived: neither fornicators, nor idolaters, nor adulterers, nor

effeminate, nor abusers of themselves with mankind. Nor thieves, nor covetous, nor drunkards, nor revilers, nor extortioners, shall inherit the kingdom of God."

1 Corinthians 6:9-10

"Meats for the belly, and the belly for meats: but God shall destroy both it and them. Now the body is not for fornication, but for the Lord; and the Lord for the body. And God hath both raised up the Lord, and will also raise up us by his own power. Know ye not that your bodies are the members of Christ? Shall I then take the members of Christ, and make them the members of an harlot? God forbid."
1 Corinthians 6:13-15

"Therefore, brethren, we are debtors, not to the flesh, to live after the flesh. For if ye live after the flesh, ye shall die: but if ye through the Spirit do mortify the deeds of the body, ye shall live."

Romans 8:12-13 (KJV)

"Stand fast therefore in the liberty wherewith Christ hath made us free, and be not entangled again with the yoke of bondage."

Galatians 5:1 (KJV)

RU TIRED?
THE REFORMERS UNANIMOUS DIFFERENCE

R U tired? If so, try RU! At Reformers Unanimous International Addictions Program, we strive to help everyone find freedom from stubborn habits and addictions introducing them to the only Truth that makes free—Jesus Christ.

But, many other people do the same type of thing. They say, "Try Jesus!" But, after you give Him a try, they are nowhere to be found. If you are going to "give Jesus a try," you must have support to strengthen you in your trials. For to "try Jesus" as they often say, is to be "tried by Jesus."

You see, life is full of trials and turmoil. It is these trials that lead many of us to find a drug of choice to avoid the reality of life. But, there is a better way! Jesus longs to save you from this world and all its various vices. He wants to not only face your trials *with* you, He wants to face your trials *for* you!

Some think religion is a crutch. Well, if something is broken, it needs a crutch to support it while it strengthens. That is what we seek to do at RU. We seek to support you as God strengthens you over your many weaknesses in life.

I don't want you to try Jesus. Rather, I want you to just stop trying! Let God do the work in your life. He has a wonderful plan for you! My co-author and friend, Dr George Crabb, and I want to reveal that wonderful plan to you in this book.

If you are attending or would like to attend one of our hundreds of meetings that are held weekly throughout the world, we will commit to support you like a crutch. After all, that is what religion is supposed to be—God's support group. God's support system and its body of believers is found within good local churches. Every RU program in America meets in a local church or is sponsored by a local church. For this reason, we can commit to you that when you come to an RU program, you will be met by people who love God, who know God, and who are willing to serve you on behalf of God.

Below is a list of ways in which we at RU will support you as God empowers you to overcome your stubborn habits or addictions. Welcome to a ministry that has as its primary purpose love and support as you gain victory over life's vices.

THE RUI MINISTRIES STUDENT SUPPORT SYSTEM

Stories of Victory: RU tired of hearing the "war stories" of people who have no real freedom in their life? **If so, try RU!** Every week, our students share how God has changed their lives through real-life, relevant stories. This weekly forty minutes of encouraging testimonies will get your weekend started off just right.

Great Teaching: RU tired of talking about problems and doing nothing about them? **If so, try RU!** Every RU class ends with a 30-minute teaching lesson that exposes valuable Bible principles that are integral to your recovery process.

Complete Curriculum: RU tired of being told what is right and not being given the tools to determine what is right? **If so, try RU!** We have one of the best comprehensive discipleship curriculums in America. It is one of the best selling, too! Thousands of people have used our curriculum to learn the Truth about addictions and Christian apathy.

Motivational Awards: RU tired of trying to find the stamina to do the right thing in the face of mounting adversity? **If so, try RU!** We will not only encourage you and help you to do the right thing, but we will also motivate you to do so. Though an award system is just a small way of doing this, it is evidence of a program that believes in acknowledging accomplishment and rewarding participation.

Free Personal Counseling: RU tired of having to get advice from people who know little about your struggles? RU tired of having to pay hourly fees to hear yourself talk? **If so, try RU!** We offer free group and individual spiritual counseling on a wide variety of topics from addiction, to marriage, finances, family, and many other areas. You will have a leader, a helper, a director, and even the pastor available as your own personal counselors during times of urgent need.

Well-Trained Local Leadership Staff: RU tired of attending programs where the leaders and volunteer workers have the same problems as you? **If so, try RU!** Our leaders have been made free from the power of sin and can openly speak about it. They do not seek anonymity. They earnestly proclaim that Jesus is the reason for their freedom, and they have been well trained to use our program and its tools to get that salvation message to you and to those whom you love.

Exciting Children's Program: RU tired of trying to find someone to help you with your child's issues while you are still trying to deal with your many issues in life? **If so, try RU!** We will not only care for your children while you attend your class, but we will entertain, teach, and develop your children. We want them to avoid the same pitfalls that ensnared many of us. They will enjoy games, prizes, snacks, play time, awards, great teaching, and many other things. Our "Kidz Club" is the weekly highlight of every child that attends.

Clean, Well-Staffed Nurseries: RU tired of programs that will not care for your little ones? **If so, try RU!** Those programs say "come as you are." But, you "are" a family; you should be able to come "as a family." If churches can offer free nurseries, then why can't an addiction program? Our clean nurseries are well staffed by volunteers of the hosting church. These volunteers have been screened and trained; and they will love your children because they love children!

Free Transportation: RU tired of trying to find a ride to places that are wanting to and waiting to help you? **If so, try RU!** We want to pick you up and will do so for almost every one of our weekly meetings, if necessary. Though some exceptions may apply, our trained drivers are here for those of you who may be without a car or license. No questions will be asked, except your address, of course!

Weekly Fellowship Time: RU tired of being alone absent of any good friends with whom you could fellowship? **If so, try RU!** RU offers its own "Happy Hour" fellowship time at the conclusion of Friday meetings. As well, our Sunday and mid-week meetings usually offer multiple opportunities to fellowship with your fellow students and leaders. Fellowship is "R" specialty; what about "U"? Then join RU! Visitors, the *RU Happy Hour* is an optional part of our Friday night class. Refreshments and food are usually served, and served well.

Residential Treatment Centers: RU tired of trying to find residential treatment that is effective and affordable? **If so, try RU!** We operate a beautiful 100-bed facility for men and a gorgeous 40-bed facility for women at our headquarters in Rockford, Illinois. This program boasts an over 90% success rate among its graduates. We are also aware of many RU type transitional homes that may be available for your use. Please visit www.reformu.com to learn more information about our homes and to download an application.

Multi-Meeting Assemblies Weekly: RU tired of not being able to find a meeting when you need one? **If so, try RU!** We offer two to three meetings every weekend and even some during the week. Plus, we offer many activities and service opportunities for our students. Please see your RU director to find the times and days of our meetings and the hosting church's service times.

Local Church Support: "I am here to tell you that **I am not tired any more.** However, if it was not for my church, I would either be dead or a dying drug addict today!" I believe, as does your hosting church's pastor, that the local church is God's support group. It is designed by God to meet the spiritual needs of all people. When the spiritual needs of people are met, then other needs fall in line and become easier to manage. As a program, we strongly encourage you to visit the church that hosts this meeting for addicted people. Something must be different about this church if they are so willing to have this program for you. Why aren't others?

In conclusion to this chapter, I want you to understand something about this book. It is a progression of truth. What that means is that we will begin to explain things to you about your drug of choice. We will teach you the physical effects of **addiction**, explain the soulical effects (which are the effects of the drug to your mind, will, and emotions), and expose the negative spiritual effects.

When we begin to expose the spiritual effects that your wrong behavior has had and will have on your life and your eternity, the truths will begin to progress from simple to understand to quite obscure. You may not quite comprehend everything you read, at least not at first. But, stay with it and gain the information. Your confidence in the truth taught may progress over time, but it is important that we explain it all right away and right here.

The three truths that will be expressed are called **justification,**

sanctification and **glorification**. Those are Old English words for modern day phenomenons. They are literal experiences that will take place in everyone's life who believes in Jesus. These three experiences are what we want you to understand, as God enables you to, that you may experience a lasting victory.

Most Christian books that are written for first-time church or class visitors only explain how one can get to heaven when they die. But, they often fail to explain how to enjoy the journey there! In these topical books on addiction recovery, Dr. Crabb and I will explain truths that make up what we call the "Hidden Life," which is our life hid IN the Life of Christ (or, HID-IN-Life). We will introduce you to a pilgrimage that will give you lasting victory over your addiction. This pilgrimage of the HID-IN-Life will bring you a peace and joy that you may have thought was not available to the inhabitants of this world.

In conclusion, be excited about this fact. The secret that has remained hidden to you that will grant you lasting sobriety is this: The life you long for is found in a Life that longs to live withIN you!

May God be with you so that you may change . . . *finally*!

Steven Curington
President and Founder
Reformers Unanimous Ministries

ACID

ACID
THE TESTIMONIES

Mary's Testimony

My experience with hallucinogens began when I was a teenager. My experience began with LSD, or, at the time, I knew it as microdot, blotter, and windowpane acid. I began with an acid known as "orange sunshine." Once it took effect, I began to laugh uncontrollably, and I saw colors and people blending in all kinds of ways. As the trip progressed, I looked into the mirror to see my face and body distorting in a way that scared me. I took the other acids in an effort to take the "ultimate" trip, sort of speaking. My last trip was with the windowpane acid, and my whole world and sense of reality was distorted. I thought I was dying, so I went and laid down in an irrigation ditch in an orange grove. A friend of mine saw me and dragged me out of the ditch. God had been drawing me to Himself for many years before this incident, but this incident was the moment God started to put the full-court press on me for salvation. When my friend dragged me out of the ditch, she started to talk to me about becoming a witch and joining a coven, at which point I said, "No, I believe in God!" Even though I appreciated her for helping me through a "bad trip," I was not about to sell my soul to the devil. Shortly, thereafter, I received Jesus Christ as my personal Savior and became involved in the Reformers Unanimous Program. My involvement in the RU program has revolutionized my way of thinking and my way of life. It has taught me so much about who I am and who Jesus Christ is. I am so thankful that my Heavenly Father has given me another opportunity to serve him.

Adam's Testimony

My first and only experience with acid started out awesome and then became scary. I was with my best friends, and one of them looked really weird to me. Her tongue was like a snake's tongue, and her head started to spin around. I truly began to freak out. I had to go into another room with other people "tripping." Another friend turned into the devil, and when I looked into the mirror, I turned into a demon. My heart started to beat real fast, and I thought I was just going to die. I finally got over my fear of my best friend and went into the room with him again. My best friend and the rest of the people there were watching the Wizard of Oz on television and everything was just unreal. I am so happy that I survived. I wanted the trip to end real badly when I saw the devil. I kept thinking I was going to die! I had to have my best friend's brother keep telling me that I was going to be fine. I can't believe I even experimented with this type of drug.

I was raised in a Christian home and have known Jesus Christ as my Savior for several years. I have dabbled here and there with certain drugs but nothing like this acid. If ever the phrase "Scared straight" applied to anyone, it was to me in this situation. After I sobered up, I confessed to my parents and my pastor what had transpired, and I also told them about all the other times I experimented with drugs. At their advice, I started to attend a Reformers Unanimous Program on Friday nights. The cool thing is that my parents go with me, and it is actually a night that we can have together, not only as a family but a night we can have together as we learn about our Heavenly Father.

I now am actually glad that I had that "bad trip." My life is so much sweeter, and my relationship with my parents is great!

Mary and Adam could not take the internal pain any longer. They saw no way to escape the pain or sense of hopelessness except through continued use of hallucinogens. Like Mary and Adam, many people of all ages and walks of life battle with the seemingly invincible problem of this addiction on a daily basis.

Does the scenario of Mary or Adam describe you or someone you love? Are you searching for answers? There are millions of people just like you or someone you know who are desperately seeking for their way out. Like Mary and Adam, many have found that way out. They were introduced to "the Way," the Lord Jesus Christ, and have joined thousands of addicts who have found freedom through this program called Reformers Unanimous (RU). RU directs people to the Truth Who makes free. I speak of the Truth named the Lord Jesus Christ. Many have come to an RU meeting, facing a combination of destructive circumstances. Many have sought help on their own, like Mary and Adam, without any long-term success. Yet, these same people are transformed as they engage in the RU curriculum and participate in its extremely supportive weekly programs.

Thousands of these individuals are now productive members of society. Collectively, they are a living testimony that there is hope for you or for those whom you love.

Yes, hallucinogens CAN be eliminated from your life. There is hope! There is freedom! And, that is the gospel TRUTH!

ACID
THE TOPIC

Each hallucinogenic user knows exactly how hallucinogens make them feel. They also recognize that the feeling it generates each time is fairly consistent. However, very few users actually know why it makes them feel this way, much less how it happens.

As with all other addictive drugs, it is amazing to learn how effective they are at masking the real root problem in a person's life. Hallucinogenic drugs actually manipulate neurotransmitters in the brain that create a false sense of well being. This sense of pleasure and calmness is, of course, only temporary. As well, it is not reality. However, we have a very great Creator who made our body to secrete these neurotransmitters, and He has ways of doing so without the pain and misery of illegal and habit-forming drugs.

NEUROTRANSMITTERS AND THEIR ROLES IN THE BODY:

- Acetylcholine: stimulates muscles, aids in sleep cycle
- Norepinephrine: similar to adrenaline, increases heart rate; helps form memories
- GABA (gamma-aminobutyric acid): prevents anxiety
- Glutamate: aids in memory formation
- Serotonin: regulates mood and emotion
- Endorphin: necessary for pleasure and pain reduction
- Dopamine: motivation; pleasure

In this chapter, Dr. George Crabb, a board certified Internal Medicine physician and member of the American Society of Addiction Medicine, will explain to us the phenomenon and feeling of this mood and mind-altering drug of choice for so many.

Mary and Adam, who we read about earlier, experienced the effects of a class of drugs called hallucinogens. Both Mary and Adam took certain types of hallucinogens called acids. They ended up seeing things that were not really there, and they both had thoughts that they would never have a normal thought again. Hallucinogenic drugs work on the body by altering the way a person thinks, feels, or experiences reality. Some of these drugs are found in nature while others are created in laboratories. While all of these drugs affect the chemicals or neurotransmitters in the brain, they all do not work the same way. The effects of each drug are slightly different even though they all change perception.

Mary and Adam took **LSD.** LSD stands for *lysergic acid diethylamide.* LSD was synthesized in the laboratory for medical purposes, but it was

quickly determined that it had no dramatic medical effects. The use of LSD can give the individual terrifying hallucinations and bizarre emotions, making the individual feel as if they are going insane. In the 1960's, many felt that hallucinogenic drugs, such as LSD, could give deep, spiritual insights. When the drug was banned, chemists in illegal laboratories synthesized LSD to sell to users. LSD is almost always ingested (taken by mouth), most commonly using blotter paper. When LSD is made, it is in crystal form. It is then dissolved in liquid, and this liquid is usually soaked up by a piece of blotter paper. The paper is then dried and cut into tiny squares, with each square being one dose. Adam took the dose by putting the square on his tongue and letting it dissolve. Sometimes the liquid is mixed with gelatin and made into thin sheets called windowpane. LSD is such a powerful drug that only a very small amount can create an intense experience, as Adam testified. LSD usually takes effect within thirty minutes of ingesting it, and the effects can last for twelve hours or longer. Physical changes come first, often causing dizziness, increased heart rate, and nausea. Within an hour, a person can begin to feel a sense of unreality and the beginnings of visual hallucinations, such as colors and lights. Time is often experienced differently while under the influence of LSD. Thus, a few seconds might feel like an hour. The experience of taking LSD or other hallucinogenic drugs is frequently called a "trip" or, as in Adam's case, a "bad trip." A person is often tired after the drug wears off. They usually have a bad headache. After a few days of taking LSD, the body builds up a tolerance. This means that a person does not experience as strong a high from the same dosage. In addition, individuals who have developed a tolerance for LSD, such as Mary, also show an increased tolerance for other hallucinogenic drugs. Tolerance is experienced with many drugs after prolonged usage, and addicts of drugs, such as cocaine and heroin, tend to cope by taking larger amounts to achieve the same high. The larger the dose of LSD, the more likely an individual will experience a "bad trip."

PCP is known as a dissociative drug. This means that it causes individuals to feel disconnected from their bodies and the world around them. Its chemical name is *phencyclidine*. Like LSD, PCP was developed by a pharmaceutical company as a legitimate drug. The scientists found that the PCP could act as an opiate, stimulant, sedative, and a hallucinogen, which is unusual since most drugs act as only one of these types. Users were affected differently depending on the size of the dose and the person's metabolism. They could either be wildly excited and energized or left in a catatonic state for hours. Others became agitated and had horrific hallucinations. Scientists wondered if they could change the chemicals in PCP just a little so that it could still work as an anesthetic without the bad side effects. These experiments gave them **ketamine**, which is similar to PCP but less powerful. Today, ketamine is used in veterinarian medicine and sometimes as an anesthetic for people.

> **HALLUCINOGEN FACT**
> A person taking LSD may "see music" or "hear colors."
> Flowers may have faces and time may seem to move differently.

Because it can cause hallucinations and bizarre sensations, physicians use it less often than other anesthetics. PCP and ketamine are highly addictive. It causes individuals to crave more and more. The combination of delusions and detachment that PCP, and to a lesser extent, ketamine, causes can make users do extremely dangerous things. Users often feel like they are indestructible and cannot be hurt. People are much more likely to die from doing crazy things while taking PCP than with any other drug. PCP is taken in several different ways. Most often, it is sprinkled on mint, oregano, parsley, or marijuana leaves and then smoked. Some times it is ingested, injected, or inhaled through the nose in powder form. Ketamine is taken in similar ways, and it is less commonly smoked. Ketamine's effects last around an hour, and the effects of PCP can last eight hours or even several days.

Other hallucinogenic drugs are **peyote** and **mescaline**. Peyote is a small cactus without any spines. The top of the cactus is covered with buttons, and these buttons are harvested for use as a hallucinogenic drug. The hallucinatory effects of peyote are similar to LSD. The main psychoactive component of peyote is mescaline. Mescaline can be created in a laboratory and, again, it will have similar hallucinatory effects as LSD.

Like peyote, **psilocybin mushrooms** have been used by native people in Mexico and Central America for thousands of years. These mushrooms contain a psychoactive compound called psilocin, which creates a less-powerful LSD-like effect. These mushrooms are called magic mushrooms or shrooms and are usually dried and eaten. Sometimes, though, the psychoactive chemicals in the mushrooms are created separately in a laboratory and sold as a white powder. In the United States, psilocybin mushrooms have become the second most popular hallucinogen after LSD.

Like Mary and Adam, many people have been using hallucinogens for centuries. The hippie-counter culture was a rebellion against a traditional culture and ways of life, and drugs, such as hallucinogens, were often a part of this rebellion.

In the late 1990's, a type of party known as a "rave" began to become popular in the United States. Raves were common in the United Kingdom and Europe a decade earlier. A rave is an all-night dance party held in a warehouse or other large, out-of-the-way buildings. Common characteristics of the rave are electronic dance music, a dark or nearly-dark building, dancing with glow sticks or LED's, and drugs. **Ecstasy** became common at raves and parties and ketamine was frequently used as well. Although ecstasy is not strictly a hallucinogen, it changes the way users see the world and can cause visual hallucinations at high doses. Ecstasy is known as MDMA. It is a difficult drug to classify. It is usually known as a club drug since it is popular at clubs and parties. Sometimes it is called an empathogen because it can produce feelings of empathy in users. Ecstasy acts as a stimulant but can have hallucinogenic effects

> **HALLUCINOGEN FACT**
> Many hallucinogenic trips are bizarre and even frightening.

at high doses. Ecstasy has led to serious medical emergencies or death, i.e., kidney failure caused by a very high body temperature.

Many people today, like Mary and Adam, are using hallucinogens. A group that monitors the future studies drug use among teenagers. In 2006 they reported that 3.4 percent of eighth graders, 6.1 percent of tenth graders, and 8.3 percent of twelfth graders had tried a hallucinogenic drug. Also, 0.9 percent of eighth graders, 1.5 percent of tenth graders, and 1.5 percent of twelfth graders had used some kind of hallucinogenic drug in the thirty days prior to the survey.

There are many dangers of hallucinogens. One of my patients told me that everything he looked at had grown rainbow edged, dancing with swirling, fractal patterns. Another young lady told me she smelled colors and tasted sounds because her senses were mixed and blended. Another teenage girl named Megan said she curled in the corner because she thought something was watching her. She thought that something terrifying was trying to find a way into her room. John watched in horror as the posters on his wall turned monster-faced and fixed their burning eyes on him. Doug felt exhausted and feared he would never be normal again. These are all different people with all different reactions to a hallucinogenic drug. The effects of hallucinogens can be extremely hard to predict. Even if a person has taken the drug many times before, they will still have a completely different experience the next time. Again, I will reiterate that hallucinogens are extremely dangerous in many ways.

Horrific complications with ketamine can be devastating for the rest of a person's life. Ketamine users become disorientated and begin to hallucinate, losing touch with their body and their identity. A ketamine user can find it difficult to move. When the effects wear

HALLUCINOGEN FACT
Many people who use hallucinogens believe it will expand their souls, allowing them to perceive and connect with the spiritual world.

off, a person usually does not remember what happened while under the influence of the ketamine. In the case of many women, ketamine has opened the door for sexual abuse and exploitation.

There are many horror stories of people committing violent murders or mutilating themselves while under the influence of PCP. LSD and other hallucinogens can sometimes trigger a complete psychological breakdown. Even after coming off the drug, many have remained paranoid, depressed, and agitated, thus, affecting the rest of their lives. Another serious consequence of LSD use is flashbacks. Those that have taken LSD in the past, even years in the past, can suddenly have a hallucinogenic experience for no apparent reason. An extreme form of flashbacks is called **hallucinogen persisting perception disorder** (HPPD). A person suffering HPPD has trouble living a normal life because of their flashbacks. The flashbacks usually only last for a minute or two and happen occasionally, but some people live with almost constant, visual hallucinations. There is absolutely no treatment available for HPPD!

Friend, regardless of where you may be in your struggle with a hallucinogen addiction, the good news is that there is life after hallucinogens. Mary and Adam found this life. For this to be accomplished in your life, there must be a change in your behavior. I want you to know that the only effective way of changing your behavior is changing the beliefs to which you hold. This will be the subject of the remainder of this book.

ALCOHOL

Kevin's Testimony

he thrill of attention is what I live for. At a young age, my athletic talent fed my pride and desire for attention. People remarked on my great talent and what I would be able to accomplish in the future. I watched as my brother played football for the University of Michigan and was visited often by college coaches. This was the attention I desired, and I began building my body and mind for my time in the limelight. The hard work paid off. My senior year I was recruited by the top universities in America. I was nominated to the high school All-American Team. My dreams were coming true. Coach Woody Hayes from Ohio State provided me with a full scholarship to play college football after my high school graduation. The sky was the limit, and I was basking in my success! Life grew even more exciting, and I played as a freshman in the Rose Bowl's national championship game. I was experiencing the world at a speed I never knew existed. It was fast, and I was famous. With stardom came a Hollywood lifestyle that I plunged head-long into. I took advantage of every experience I was offered. However, in three short years my success fizzled out, and my football career at Ohio State University ended.

Next, I dove into a business career with the expectation of receiving great affirmation for the things I would be doing. However, I carried with me the alcohol and drugs from college. I had learned the art of manipulation and was lying to carry out my desires and remain in full control. Praise came but it was not fulfilling. In 1991, I married my high school sweetheart. We had two children, owned two homes, and I had all the toys I ever wanted. I had dreamed of this lifestyle and drove myself until I became a successful businessman with no desires unfulfilled. Then, I was drawn to the political scene, and the power that certain positions held. I became the council president. My pride had grown to the highest level of my life, but it was not enough to have a beautiful family as well as a financial, political, and professional success. I was coaching football for my children and head of my church council. I had the freedom and respect of everyone I came in contact with except myself. I began to self destruct, which led to my divorce in 2001. I lost my family, homes, political career, and everyone's respect. I was alone and had no peace. My only friend was a bottle of vodka. I tried to rebuild and remarry but that, too, ended in a divorce.

On December 23, 2005 my family introduced me to Reformers Unanimous International. I was saved on Christmas Day and baptized on New Year's Eve. Since then, I have found the true love of people and experienced the grace and mercy of our Savior, Jesus Christ. God has used this program to break me down as a man of pride and slowly develop me into a man of God. After two years of recovery, I work for Reformers Unanimous and use my skills to reach people and tell them of Christ. I am also in charge of the alumni association for the Reformers Unanimous Schools of Discipleship. I believe God has placed me here to humble me so I may learn to love God and others and to serve God and others. I want to teach other men about my life's experiences in finding the Lord. He brings perfect peace. I have a wonderful relationship today with my Lord, my family, and my children. I am glad I never quit or gave up. God has taught me to stand still and wait for Him to calm the storms of life. To God be the glory!

Kevin could not take the internal pain any longer. He saw no way to escape the pain or sense of hopelessness except through continued use of alcohol. Like Kevin, many people of all ages and walks of life battle with the seemingly invincible problem of alcohol addiction on a daily basis.

Does the scenario of Kevin describe you or someone you love? Are you searching for answers? There are millions of people just like you or someone you know who are desperately seeking for their way out. Like Kevin, many have found that way out. They were introduced to "the Way," the Lord Jesus Christ, and have joined thousands of addicts who have found freedom through this program called **Reformers Unanimous (RU)**. RU directs people to the Truth Who makes free. I speak of the Truth named the Lord Jesus Christ. Many have come to an RU meeting, facing a combination of destructive circumstances. Many have sought help on their own, like Kevin, without any long-term success. Yet, these same people are transformed as they engage in the RU curriculum and participate in its extremely supportive weekly programs.

Thousands of these individuals are now productive members of society. Collectively, they are a living testimony that there is hope for you or for those whom you love.

Yes, alcohol CAN be eliminated from your life. There is hope! There is freedom! And, that is the gospel TRUTH!

ALCOHOL
THE TOPIC

ach alcohol user knows exactly how alcohol makes them feel. They also recognize that the feeling it generates each time is fairly consistent. However, very few drinkers actually know why it makes them feel this way, much less how it happens.

As with all other addictive drugs, it is amazing to learn how effective they are at masking the real root problem in a person's life. Alcohol actually manipulates neurotransmitters in the brain that create a false sense of well being. This sense of pleasure and calmness is, of course, only temporary. As well, it is not reality. However, we have a very great Creator who made our body to secrete these neurotransmitters, and He has ways of doing so without the pain and misery of alcohol abuse.

NEUROTRANSMITTERS AND THEIR ROLES IN THE BODY:

- Acetylcholine: stimulates muscles, aids in sleep cycle
- Norepinephrine: similar to adrenaline, increases heart rate; helps form memories
- GABA (gamma-aminobutyric acid): prevents anxiety
- Glutamate: aids in memory formation
- Serotonin: regulates mood and emotion
- Endorphin: necessary for pleasure and pain reduction
- Dopamine: motivation; pleasure

In this chapter, Dr. George Crabb, a board certified Internal Medicine physician and member of the American Society of Addiction Medicine, will explain to us the phenomenon and feeling of this mood and mind-altering drug of choice for so many.

Kevin, who we read about earlier, experienced the effect of alcohol, which is a chemical produced by the fermentation of a starch-based substance. There are different types of alcohol, such as ethyl alcohol (ethanol) used for consumption, butyl alcohol (butanol) used in adhesives and varnishes, and methyl alcohol (methanol or wood alcohol) used in industrial solvents. During the prohibition years, some people mixed wood alcohol with ethyl alcohol which led to irreversible blindness. A fourth type of alcohol is isopropyl alcohol, which is rubbing alcohol. This type of alcohol is used as a disinfectant and also as an ingredient in colognes and perfumes. Lastly is ethylene glycol, which is antifreeze and the most deadly of all the alcohols to ingest.

Alcoholic beverages depend on a chemical change occurring in a substance's molecular structure through a process called fermentation. Fermentation consumes the starch substance and carbon dioxide and ethyl alcohol are released. Beer is one of the oldest alcoholic beverages in the world today. It is largely produced by the fermentation of barley or rice. Alcohol has been a part of our history for thousands of years. The first mention of drunkenness is mentioned in Genesis 9:21 regarding an episode in Noah's life. One thing is certain and that is the impact alcohol has had on the world. The negative consequences are illustrated in the story of Noah (Genesis 9:20-27). Many look at the consumption of alcohol as a right of passage. Others, like Kevin, initially looked at consumption of alcohol as a recreational beverage, not contemplating the tremendous side effects that come with the ingestion of this drug.

A mother brought her teenage son to my office so that I could address with him the consequences of drinking alcohol. This young man told me that the reason he started drinking alcohol was the following: "I have always been shy. In the past, I have felt ignored and left out. But, as soon as I drank the beer, everything seemed wonderful. I was no longer shy. I felt like I could talk to anybody, and it seemed like everyone enjoyed being with me. Other people finally found it fun to be with me." This young man, as well as Kevin, perceived alcohol to be beneficial because it made him more at ease in social situations. But, the effects of the alcohol do not stop there! The alcohol becomes a problem, not only for them but for all those around them. There is absolutely no doubt that alcohol changes an individual's behavior. To understand how it accomplishes this, we must first understand how alcohol works on the body.

When Kevin had an alcoholic drink, his stomach would absorb about twenty percent of the alcohol. The remaining eighty percent of the alcohol was absorbed by his small intestines. How quickly Kevin's body absorbed alcohol depended upon the following:

1. The amount of alcohol he drank.
2. The type of drink (carbonated beverages speed up the absorption of alcohol).

3. The amount of food in his stomach (food slows down the absorption of alcohol).
4. The individual's size, weight, and gender. (Women are affected more quickly because they are generally smaller than men.)

As the alcohol was absorbed from Kevin's stomach and small intestinal tract, the alcohol would then enter his blood stream and dissolve in the water component of the blood. The alcohol then traveled through his body entering and dissolving in each tissue (except fat) of his body. Once the alcohol has entered the tissues of the body, its effects begin to be experienced. What effects an individual such as Kevin would feel depends on the blood alcohol concentration (BAC). Most people, including Kevin, begin to feel the effects of alcohol between ten and twenty minutes after taking the first drink. There is typically an elevation in mood followed by a calmness and sedative effect. As the alcohol is coursing through the blood system of Kevin, his kidneys and lungs would eliminate a small percentage, but his liver would start the breakdown process of the majority of the alcohol through a chemical process called oxidation. The alcohol in Kevin's blood system would track into his brain, thus, crossing the blood-brain barrier. Alcohol is a depressant, which means it affects mental and physical functioning. When the alcohol reached Kevin's brain, it affected his brain's complex communication system by acting on its nerve cells called neurons. Alcohol, just like any other mind and mood-altering drug, affects the brain by manipulating the body's own natural neurotransmitters. In the case of alcohol, the neurotransmitter involved is gamma-aminobutyric acid (GABA), which is an inhibitor. The alcohol in Kevin's brain increased the effects of GABA, causing his actions to become sluggish. Alcohol also weakens the neurotransmitter glutamine, which is an excitatory neurotransmitter. So, the alcohol in Kevin's brain not only increased the effectiveness of GABA, which is an inhibitor, but also weakened the effect of the excitatory neurotransmitter glutamine, both with the end result of feeling sluggish. As Kevin's blood alcohol concentration (BAC) increased, the effect on his brain increased. His cerebral cortex, the part of the brain responsible for processing sensory information (thought processing, consciousness, and initiating voluntary muscular movements) felt the effects of the alcohol first. The alcohol depressed his behavioral inhibitory centers, causing him to become more talkative and less shy (like the teenager I talked about earlier). It also slows down his processing of sensory information, which causes problems seeing, touching, and tasting and inhibits thought processes leading to impaired judgment. Kevin's limbic system would be the next part of his brain to feel the effect of alcohol. This is the area of the brain that controls emotions and memory. Kevin, being under the influence of this drug, had exaggerated emotional states, such as rage, extreme sadness, and loss of memory. Kevin's cerebellum would be the next part of the brain affected by the alcohol. When the cerebellum is affected by the influence of alcohol, Kevin began to lose motor skills. The cerebellum controls fine movements, tasks that would normally be completed with no difficulty, such as touching a finger to the nose with closed eyes. Kevin's movements became jerky, and with higher levels of blood alcohol concentration, he would become uncoordinated, finding walking difficult if not impossible. As the alcohol systematically finds its way through different parts of the brain, the medulla (brain stem) would be next in line to feel the effects of alcohol. The medulla controls involuntary functions, such as breathing, heart rate, consciousness, and temperature. When the effects of the alcohol reached Kevin's medulla, he began to feel sleepy. And, if the blood alcohol concentration is high enough, the individual may pass out. When an individual has consumed a large amount of alcohol, thus, having a high blood alcohol concentration, the respiration rate can become very slow, and in fact, individuals can stop breathing. I have witnessed this many times in the emergency room. The heart rate can slow dramatically, causing the individual's blood pressure and body temperature to drop to dangerously low levels, which are potentially fatal. The effects of alcohol are exacerbated by tranquilizers, which cause profound respiratory depression followed by comma and death.

We must also realize, although the main effect of alcohol is on the brain, it is not limited to the brain. Alcohol, even in the smallest amounts, promotes aging of the skin. As people continue in their addiction to alcohol, they begin replacing nutritional calories with non-nutritional calories found in alcohol. The malabsorption process occurs, which leads to multiple vitamin B deficiencies. The above causes:

- Brittle Hair
- Puffy Skin
- Cracked Lips
- Broken Vein Appearance
- Increased Acne Breakouts
- Increased Blood Flow to Skin (causing excess sweating and flushing of face)

Kevin, as he continued in his alcohol addiction, experienced symptoms of heartburn. Alcohol can irritate the lining of the esophagus and the stomach, causing stomach ulcerations. Alcohol also increases the risk of cancers of the mouth, esophagus, stomach, and intestines. But, of course, the liver suffers the most damage since it is the primary organ in the body where alcohol is broken down. Cirrhosis is a liver disease often found in people addicted to alcohol, and Cirrhosis can lead to liver failure, which is fatal.

Another effect on the body from alcoholic Cirrhosis is called esophageal varisees. Esophageal varisees are varicose veins within the lining of the esophagus. These have a tendency to break open and when this occurs, massive hemorrhage (bleeding) occurs. If not dealt with immediately, death is the end result. Alcohol also causes reduction of blood flow to the muscles. Kevin, being a conditioned athlete, would suffer from severe muscle cramping, secondary to his alcohol use.

Despite all of the above negative consequences of alcohol, Kevin believed the lie that alcohol was a necessity to his life, something he could not life without. It is estimated that in America today there are 17.6 million adults that have the same thought process as Kevin.

Kevin has testified to me personally that he had unbelievable cravings to drink alcohol. He went on to say that he would need to drink greater amounts of alcohol in order to "get high." Kevin stated that the craving for a drink of alcohol became the overwhelming motivation for getting through the day. As Kevin and others continue in their alcohol addiction, changes in their brain chemistry occur. Long-term alcohol use eventually depletes the brain's supply of the neurotransmitters dopamine and serotonin, leaving the individual depressed with little or no motivation and pleasure.

As Kevin continued in his alcohol addiction, he stated that he started to drink to get relief from the problems and stress of his daily life. He needed more and more alcohol to feel drunk. He experienced blackouts where he was unable to remember events or blocks of time that happened while drinking. He began to hide alcohol in certain places of his home, vehicle, and place of business. As already mentioned, he began to think more and more about alcohol to where it was the consuming thought of every moment, and he started to plan activities around drinking.

Withdrawal from alcohol is a difficult, dangerous, and potentially deadly process. These symptoms can occur just several hours from the individual's last drink. Kevin experienced some of the following withdrawal symptoms:

- Tremulousness
- Fever / Sweating
- Rapid Heart Beat / Palpitations
- Increased or Decreased Blood Pressure
- Extreme, Aggressive Behavior
- Auditory and Visual Hallucinations
- Seizure Activity
- DTs (Delirium Tremens which develop 2 days after the last drink of alcohol)

I must reiterate to the reader that alcohol withdrawal can be potentially fatal. In light of this, medical attention is a necessity.

The dangers of alcohol addiction are enormous. It is estimated that each year approximately 100,000 deaths can be attributed to drinking, either directly or indirectly. An individual who is addicted to alcohol and continues in that lifestyle can expect to have their life cut short by 10-15 years. The tragedy is that the dangers go beyond the alcohol addict and affect those around him. Alcohol can kill in so many different ways. Those who are addicted to alcohol have a higher rate of death from:

- Injury
- Violence
- Some Caners (mentioned earlier)

They have higher risk for alcohol-related medical disorders, such as:
- Pancreatitis
- Upper Gastrointestinal Bleeding
- Nerve Damage (Neuropathy)
- Alcoholic-Cardiomyopathy (weakening of heart muscle)
- Korsakoff Syndrome (A condition brought about by the deficiency of thiamin, one of the B vitamins. This syndrome causes significant short-term memory impairment. Individuals with this type of syndrome often confabulate to fill in memory gaps.)

Those that are addicted to alcohol that may require some form of surgery have an increased risk of post-operative complications, including:
- Infections
- Bleeding
- Slow Wound Healing

It is also a well known fact that alcohol is a factor in more than one-half of all motor vehicle accidents. According to a 2001 study quoted on Reuter's Health, alcohol is a factor in 25 percent of people who commit suicide. This study also went on to demonstrate that alcohol was a factor in almost 70 percent of all murders. Alcohol also exacerbates domestic violence. Children of alcohol-addicted parents have less success at school. They are more depressed, have fewer friends, and have lower self esteem than their peers. Women who continue in their addiction while pregnant run the risk of giving birth to a baby with fetal alcohol syndrome (FAS). Babies born with FAS can have some or most of the following characteristics:

- Facial Deformities
- Intellectual Impairment
- Memory Problems
- Delayed Development
- Impaired Motor Skills
- Hyperactivity
- Neurosensory Hearing Loss
- Learning Disabilities
- Impaired Visual/Spacial Skills

ALWAYS REMEMBER: The above are conditions that last a lifetime!

The devastation that Kevin and others have realized in their lives is a real problem for teenagers in our society today. There are many teenagers that start drinking alcohol because they like the way it makes them feel. It gives them that temporary relief from the "stress of life." In our society, drinking alcohol seems almost normal for the adolescent, but the consequences are very serious. According to the national survey on drug use and health in 2002-2004, more than 18 million individuals between the ages of 12-17 admitted to being dependent on alcohol during the previous year. Reasons that teenagers drink are as follows:

EVERYBODY ELSE DOES

- Promoted by Television, Internet, and Magazines
ESCAPE FROM STRESS OF LIFE

- Extreme Disappointment

- **Depression**
- **Loneliness**

REBELLION

- **Angry (no release of bottled-up anger)**
- **Act Out Aggression**

As we have noted, addiction to alcohol is a major cause of disease, disability, and death in the United States as well as world-wide. One of the many reasons that alcohol is so destructive is that it is commonly associated with other drug use. Addition to alcohol occurs commonly with addiction to narcotics. For example, up to 89% of cocaine addicts are also addicted to alcohol. Abuse of other psychostimulants, sedatives (e.g., benzodiazepines, barbiturates, and marijuana), and hallucinogenic drugs also occur commonly against a background of alcohol addiction. Alcohol is a major tool that Satan uses to unravel the basic fabric of our society.

All that Kevin and the other millions of individuals in our society today are looking for is help to heal the hurt that lives down deep within them.

Friend, regardless of where you may be in your struggle with alcohol addiction, the good news is that there is life after alcohol. Kevin found this life. For this to be accomplished in your life, there must be a change in your behavior. I want you to know that the only effective way of changing your behavior is changing the beliefs to which you hold. This will be the subject of the remainder of this book.

COCAINE

COCAINE
The Testimonies

Katrina's Testimony

I was raised in a good, non-Christian home with parents who encouraged my sister and me to be strong and successful. My parents divorced when I was fourteen, and that was a major turning point in my life. At fifteen, I started drinking and experimenting with drugs. I would occasionally drink during the week but much harder on the weekends. I was able to maintain good grades, so no one caught on. I began hanging out with an older crowd of mostly dropouts and ex-cons. They made me feel accepted. Adopting their lifestyle of drinking, drugs, and punk music, I wore pink and green hair, cut-up jeans, combat boots, and had multiple piercing and tattoos.

As time elapsed, I moved on to harder drugs and more addictions. Graduating from high school, after being voted class rebel and having lived a double life, I won a scholarship to a private college. At the college, I began using speed to stay awake to study, work, and party. My life began to spiral out of control. Drugs consumed my mind, and I hung out with drug dealers and criminals. I finally dropped out of college two months prior to graduation.

Like many, thinking my problem was the drugs and the city in which I resided, I tried moving. Over the next ten years, not understanding the root of my problem, I moved often. I lived in numerous states as well as in Zimbabwe, Africa. Finally, I moved to Cleveland, Ohio where I spent the next eleven years addicted to cocaine and heroine.

Well, besides the enormous drug addiction, I began to face legal problems. I was arrested seven times in six months for drug offences. I was given probation and also a treatment plan. I was court-ordered to attend AA, NA, and CA meetings, but I still ran with the bad crowd, which, of course, led to my using drugs again. Justifying my choices, I blamed society, my parents, and God. I soon violated my probation and ended up jobless, homeless, and pregnant. I so desperately wanted to get out of the life I was leading, but I could not break the chains that were holding me so tight.

Even though I did not know God on a personal basis, I prayed that He would make it all end. In the meantime, all of my drug friends were either dying or going to prison.

Two days after the birth of my son, Gabriel, I went to jail. Through this experience, though, I knew that God had saved my life. Two weeks later, my son's father, Wayne, also went to jail. We both spent the next six months behind bars.

The baby's father, Wayne, was saved at the age of ten through the bus ministry at Cleveland Baptist Church. Just prior to the both of us going to jail, we were standing on a street corner when a man stopped his car and handed us a tract from Cleveland Baptist Church. As we both stood there, we knew that we needed to go to church and even talked about attending Cleveland Baptist Church. As I said earlier, I had prayed that God would make it all end, and He was working in the background answering my prayer. Once Wayne and I were in jail, we started writing to each other. I, then, realized my need and was saved right there in jail in January 2001. We both promised each other that we would go to church as soon as we were released from jail.

Well, after released from jail, I kept that promise and was in church the Sunday following my release. At church is where I noticed a brochure for Reformers Unanimous. Right away I knew that God wanted me to attend. Wayne and I attended the RU program the day after he was released from jail. Everything that the secular programs could not do, RU and the Lord did! Wayne and I started rebuilding our lives, and we got married on August 17, 2001. We both stayed faithful to church and the RU program, but Wayne made some decisions that took our lives in a different direction. He owed his own business and decided to open another store. However, he started renting a storefront in his old stomping grounds, which was a major drug area. I immediately disagreed with his decision, but he assured me that he could withstand the temptation. Well, he could not! Soon, he was getting high and was back in Satan's snare.

On the morning of October 27, 2001, I woke up and did not see or hear Wayne. I knew that something was wrong. As I began to look for him in the house, I found him lying on the floor in the bathroom, his body cold and lifeless. Wayne had died there some two to three hours earlier. My world began shattering around me. But, even during those dark, lonely days, God was still with me. Gene and Diane Piazza, our RU director and his wife, took me into their home, and God gave me the strength to continue on. I know now that God took Wayne home because of his disobedience, and if he had continued on that path, it would have destroyed our son, Gabriel, and me as well.

Well, now it has been five years, and the Lord has blessed me in countless ways. I have full custody of my son, and he attends our church's Christian school. The Lord has given me an excellent job with a top national accounting firm. This is another miracle because they know of my criminal background. I have a nice home and all of my basic needs are met. Sometimes I remember back to the times when I was hungry, cold, tired, confused, and addicted. By remembering those times, I rejoice in how far God has brought me. God brought a special man into my life. We are now married, and he is a father to my son. Dennis and I were married in 2002 during an RU conference at our church. We have recently won custody of my husband's thirteen-year-old son, and we look forward to seeing God bless his life.

I know that my calling is to share my story with the addicted. Hopefully, by doing this, I can help them avoid the pain and hard lessons I had to endure. Most of all, I want to share with them the Jesus Christ is the ONLY WAY to true peace and freedom.

Brian's Testimony

I grew up in Cleveland, Ohio and began running the streets at a very young age. I was always in trouble at school, with the neighbors, my family, and even the police. I eventually ended up in prison with a five-year sentence for vandalism.

While incarcerated, I heard the gospel for the very first time. Well, it did not take a thirty-minute sermon to convince me that I was a sinner and on my way to hell. That day in September, I got saved! Now, I wish I could have lived a good, Christian life from that point on, but, unfortunately, it did not work out that way. Cocaine, alcohol, and the party atmosphere consumed me. This, of course, hindered me from growing spiritually in any way. I was bound to a world of addiction with no grasp of how to find freedom from it or the damage it was doing to my life.

In September 2002, about eleven years after being saved, a friend told me about a Bible-based addiction program called Reformers Unanimous.

He explained that it was very different from the other self-help groups in that it was ordained by God and rooted in Scripture. After attending my first RU meeting, I knew that this was where the Lord wanted me to be. A couple of weeks later, I became a member of the church that hosted our meetings. Joining the church and attending the RU meetings are what really stimulated me to grow as a Christian. However, as I was attending church and the meetings, I was going through a messy divorce, had my driver's license revoked, was unemployed, homeless, and in poor health.

Well, today I have experienced God's great mercy! I am happily married to a beautiful, godly woman. I am also gainfully employed, and my health is getting better and better each day. But, most of all, my relationship with the Lord Jesus Christ has developed more than in any other area in my life. I am currently involved in Sunday school, an usher in the church, and a student at our church's Bible college.

If you are struggling with an addiction, or similar circumstances, you should consider the truth found in Isaiah 55:7 – *"Let the wicked forsake his way, and the unrighteous man his thoughts: and let him return unto the LORD, and he will have mercy upon him; and to our God, for he will abundantly pardon."*

Katrina and Brian could not take the internal torment any longer. They both saw no way to escape the pain or sense of hopelessness except through continued use of cocaine. Like Katrina and Brian, many people of all ages and walks of life battle with the seemingly invincible problem of cocaine addiction on a daily basis.

Do the scenarios of Katrina or Brian describe you or someone you love? Are you searching for answers? There are millions of people just like you or someone you know who are desperately seeking for their way out. Like Katrina and Brian, many have found that way out. They were introduced to "the Way," the Lord Jesus Christ, and have joined thousands of addicts who have found freedom through this program called **Reformers Unanimous (RU)**. RU directs people to the Truth Who makes free. I speak of the Truth named the Lord Jesus Christ. Many have come to an RU meeting, facing a combination of destructive circumstances. Many have sought treatment, like Katrina, without any long-term success. Yet, these same people are transformed as they engage in the RU curriculum and participate in its extremely supportive weekly programs.

Thousands of these individuals are now productive members of society. Collectively, they are a living testimony that there is hope for you or for those whom you love.

Yes, cocaine CAN be eliminated from your life. There is hope! There is freedom! And, that is the gospel TRUTH!

COCAINE
THE TOPIC

Each cocaine user knows exactly how cocaine makes them feel. They also recognize that the feeling it generates each time is fairly consistent. However, very few users actually know why it makes them feel this way, much less how it happens.

As a former cocaine addict myself, I was amazed to learn how effective this drug was at masking the real root problem in my life. Cocaine actually stimulates **neurotransmitters** in the brain that create a false sense of enjoyment. This sense of pleasure is, of course, only temporal. As well, it is not reality. However, we have a very great Creator who made our body to secrete these **neurotransmitters,** and He has ways of doing so without the pain and misery of illegal and destructive habit forming drugs.

In this chapter, Dr. George Crabb, a board certified Internal Medicine physician and member of the American Society of Addiction Medicine, will explain to us the phenomenon and feeling of this mood and mind altering drug of choice for so many.

Katrina and Brian, whom we read about in chapter two, experienced the effects of a chemical found in the plant, *Erythroxylum coca*, which is native to South America. We know this drug as COCAINE. Cocaine is one of the world's most powerful stimulants of natural origin. It is a natural pesticide that helps keep the *coca* plant alive.

To understand the effects of cocaine on Katrina and Brian, we shall first look at how it worked on their brain. Cocaine has a powerful impact on the brain's functions. Cocaine stimulates a group of chemicals called neurotransmitters. Because of this stimulation, Katrina and Brian enjoyed the effects of this elevation of neurotransmitters in their brains through experiences of euphoria, decreased appetite, increased alertness, and an increased ability to concentrate.

Neurotransmitters (serotonin, norepinephrine, dopamine, and acetylcholine) are messengers between different nerve cells in the brain.

Cocaine increases the amounts of these neurotransmitters released in the brain, thus exciting the nerve endings and sending out even more signals. Depending upon which neurotransmitter is effected, this can make the cocaine user feel excited, powerful, and full of energy.

As witnessed in the earlier testimonies, we can see the effect of increased serotonin in the brain. Serotonin plays an important role in controlling the body's internal clock. Body temperature, sleep cycle, and appetite are all affected by serotonin. Katrina can testify that the increased levels of serotonin because of cocaine use made her experience total appetite loss for days.

Cocaine use also increases the neurotransmitter norepinephrine, which produces a state of shock. Norepinephrine helps regulate a proper response to emergency. It prepares the body to fight or escape (*The Fight or Flight Response*). Brian can testify that with the increased levels of norepinephrine in his brain, it made him feel, at the time, more energetic, and less hungry. And, because norepinephrine widens the passages in the lungs allowing more oxygen to enter the body, he would feel stronger and have a sense of invincibility. The "rush" and "excitement" that cocaine gives to the user is secondary to the stimulation of norepinephrine in the brain. The other neurotransmitter that cocaine increases the level in the brain is dopamine. Dopamine is related to the "reward" system. Dopamine reinforces the feelings achieved during pleasurable experiences, such as laughing, eating, exercising, or work. Cocaine directly activates these same circuits and helps to essentially condition or stamp in behaviors that are not only necessary for survival, but behaviors that can be highly destructive, such as crime and deception. Katrina and Brian both became involved with such destructive, compulsive, male adaptive behavior because of the effect that the increased surge of dopamine in their brain had on them as a result of their cocaine use. This led both of these individuals, as well as many others, into a life of crime and incarceration.

NEUROTRANSMITTERS AND THEIR ROLES IN THE BODY:

- Acetylcholine: stimulates muscles, aids in sleep cycle
- Norepinephrine: similar to adrenaline, increases heart rate; helps form memories
- GABA (gamma-aminobutyric acid): prevents anxiety
- Glutamate: aids in memory formation
- Serotonin: regulates mood and emotion
- Endorphin: necessary for pleasure and pain reduction

Once cocaine is broken down by a user's system, the intense surge of neurotransmitters halts, and the normal production of neurotransmitters is reduced. After experiencing unnaturally high levels of activity, the brain now experiences unnaturally low levels of activity, which leads to lethargy, loss of self-confidence, and devastatingly deep depression. This is referred to as "coming down" or "crashing."

One of the most devastating effects of cocaine is noticed when the cocaine is broken down in the user's body. The cocaine increases the concentration of neurotransmitters in one's brain. Therefore, the normal baseline production of neurotransmitters is reduced, resulting in the "crashing" effects. The post-cocaine lows drive the user to only remember the initial rush or the sense of euphoria originally experienced from cocaine. This leads to the severe unhappiness and crippling addiction, as cocaine becomes the only escape for the neurotransmitter-deficient abuser.

There are several forms of cocaine to which individuals become addicted. Katrina and Brian, like most of the other cocaine addicts in our society, are addicted to cocaine hydrochloride (cocaine powder). This is the most common form of cocaine and is the one most frequently associated with cocaine use in the media. More street names for cocaine powder are bad rock, bazooka, beam, Bernice, big C, blast, blizzard, blow, and snowstorm. Cocaine hydrochloride (or cocaine powder) has a chunk-like texture and is off-white to pink in color. It is very stable, and because of its stability, it is possible to drink, inject, or snort it. Cocaine hydrochloride (or cocaine powder) is frequently diluted with other substances known as adulterates. Baking soda is the most commonly used adulterate of cocaine hydrochloride, but many substances can be used, some more dangerous than others. By "cutting" cocaine with these additional substances, cocaine dealers are able to charge more money for less pure cocaine. These adulterates expose the user to a wide range of dangers.

Both Katrina and Brian could also tell you that the other form of cocaine widely used in society is crack cocaine. Crack cocaine is produced by heating cocaine powder in a baking soda solution until the water has evaporated, creating a rock. When the rock of cocaine is heated, it tends to crackle, giving it its name "crack cocaine." Crack is most often smoked. It offers the user an intense, temporary high that leaves them craving more. The other form of cocaine that is available is free-base cocaine. Again, most cocaine addicts, such as Katrina and Brian, used cocaine powder or crack cocaine. Free-base cocaine is extremely addictive but dangerous to make. Many individuals have died or have been severely disabled in the process of making free-base cocaine.

Katrina and Brian lived in this powerful, psycho-stimulant world of cocaine use. Their central nervous systems were repeatedly bombarded by increased levels of neurotransmitters because of their continued use of cocaine. This stimulation made their thoughts and actions seem faster as though their brains and bodies had been put into fast forward. Katrina and Brian would tell you that this sought-after sensation was originally pleasurable, but they would be quick to confess that there is a very steep price to pay for this so-called pleasure. Distorted thinking, errors in judgment, and sometimes violence become part of the consequences of such choices.

Continuing to use cocaine sends the central nervous system into a vicious, downward spiral of addiction. It creates a desire that can only be satisfied by more cocaine abuse and destroys, rather than creates, any sense of permanent satisfaction. Sadly, most cocaine users have reported psychological addictions from the first hit.

As Brian slipped deeper and deeper into the addictive lifestyle with cocaine, changes started to slowly happen in his life. His body began to adapt to the increasingly familiar presence of cocaine. His body adjusted to the increased level of neurotransmitters by minimizing the amounts of neurotransmitters naturally produced. Less available neurotransmitters in his brain made him less able to experience pleasure from normal activities and less able to experience pleasure from the drug the next time he used it. Thus, Brian needed more cocaine to get high. His system was developing a tolerance to the drug's effects. Brian needed more hits, more frequently, with less time in between for his body to adjust its neurotransmitter production to normal levels.

Brian became, at times, maniacal. His life began to center around crack cocaine without regard for food, sleep, or safety. All three of these necessities of life became irrelevant to him for they failed to supply any pleasure. But, just like everyone else, Brian experienced depression and melancholy after cocaine use.

Katrina and Brian were enjoying some of the short-term affects of cocaine use. Even after their first use of cocaine, these effects were apparent in their lives. They felt euphoric, energetic, talkative, more sociable, and mentally alert, especially to the sensation of sight, sound, and touch.

In Katrina's case, it also produced anorexia (lack of appetite). Brian found that the cocaine helped him perform simple physical and intellectual tasks more quickly. As the cocaine entered their systems, their blood vessels constricted, their pupils dilated, their core body temperature increased, their heart rate increased, and their blood pressure increased.

These physiological responses are a recipe for disaster. Death can occur and, in fact, can occur the first time an individual uses cocaine. Cocaine-related deaths are often a result of cardiac arrest or seizure activity followed by respiratory arrest.

I have experienced in my medical practice those individuals who have used large amounts of cocaine in the attempt to intensify their high. They arrive in the emergency room with bizarre, erratic, and violent behavior. I find them experiencing tremors, vertigo (dizziness), muscle twitching, and an extreme sense of paranoia. Cardiac arrhythmias, increased blood pressure, elevated temperature, chest pain, nausea, blurred vision, seizures, and coma are also well-known results of cocaine, which I have witnessed time and time again.

Unfortunately, we in the medical field see death as a result of cocaine all too often. I experienced, first hand, the devastation that cocaine can have on an individual when I was an intern at a hospital in Detroit, Michigan.

While working a night shift in the emergency room, a car drove up to the emergency room entrance. The back door flew open, and a young man's body dropped out while the car sped away. The young man, only nineteen years of age, was quickly brought into the emergency room and evaluated by myself as well as other physicians present. It was deemed that the patient was significantly intoxicated with cocaine. His heart and lungs were failing, and he had to be put on total life support.

Over the next three days, this young man developed multi-system organ failure. One after another, his organs began to shut down. During this time, none of his friends visited his bedside in the ICU. The only individual that I ever saw sitting at this young man's bedside was his mother. Her face was buried in her hands, and I could hear her praying and weeping over her son. After three days of attempting to support this young man's life, he passed away. There, in that ICU, I stood, for the first time, over the body of a 19 year old man whose life was ended by cocaine.

This event has been seared in my memory. I have since cared for other individuals who have died because of their cocaine use. In many of these cases, their cocaine use was combined with alcohol use. There is a potentially dangerous interaction between cocaine and alcohol. Taken in combination, the two drugs are converted by the body to coca ethylene. Coca ethylene has a longer duration of action in the brain and is more toxic than either drug alone. It is noteworthy that the mixture of cocaine and alcohol is the most common two-drug combination that results in drug-related deaths.

I am often asked by parents or other concerned family members, "What are some of the signs to suggest cocaine use?" I give them the following information, but I also reiterate to them that this is not an exhaustive list. Signs to suggest that someone is using cocaine are as follows:

- Red Eyes
- Running Nose; Frequent Sniffing
- Changes in Eating Habits (loss of weight)
- Changes in Sleeping Habits (sleeps all day; up all night)
- Changes in Friends and Groups of Different Ages
- Changes in Behavior
- Reduction in Grades at School
- Skipping School
- Missing Days of Work
- Losing a Job
- Frequently Needing Money
- Stealing Money to Support the Cocaine Habit
- Losing Interest in Things One Used To Do
- Acting Withdrawn or Depressed (isolation)
- Careless About Personal Appearance

There are dangers of maternal cocaine use. Katrina is now aware of the significant risk she placed her unborn child in as she continued with her cocaine use during her pregnancy. The unborn child of a mother addicted to cocaine faces an array of potential dangers before entering the world. Children born to a cocaine-abusing mother deal with the following:

- Premature Deliveries
- Lower Birth Weights
- Smaller Head Circumferences

- Shorter in Length

These children often face subtle but significant challenges throughout their development:

- Less-than-average Cognitive Performances
- Information Processing Difficulties

These are all challenges to a child's education and can severely inhibit growth, both physically and psychologically.

Cocaine also caused biological changes in the brains of Katrina and Brian. Because of these biological changes, cocaine withdrawal is a very serious issue. As they withdrew from cocaine, they experienced the following:

- Agitation
- Depression
- Craving for Drug
- Extreme Fatigue
- Anxiety
- Angry Outbursts
- Lack of Motivation
- Nausea and Vomiting
- Tremors
- Irritability
- Muscle Pain
- Disturbed Sleep Patterns

Please remember: The above list is not an exhaustive list.

Ask Katrina or Brian, or anyone else that has withdrawn from cocaine, about the effects. They will, without exception, describe a nightmare.

Friend, regardless of where you may be at this time in your struggle with cocaine addiction, the good news is that there is life after cocaine! Katrina and Brian have found this life!

For this to be accomplished in your life, there must be a change in your behavior. I want you to know that the only effective way of changing your behavior is changing the beliefs to which you hold. This will be the subject of the remainder of this book.

CUTTING

CUTTING
THE TESTIMONIES

John's Testimony

Hello, my name is John. I began to cut myself when I was about ten years old. At first, I did not realize what I was doing. One day I was very angry at my parents for not letting me to do something, and I began to scratch my arms until I felt the blood come out. Somehow, this made me feel really good. I guess it was a release of all the pain I had hidden deep in my life. At that time, I thought I had found a new friend, and therefore, I continued to seek out his companionship. I began by cutting my feet and ankles, and then I started cutting my thighs. It helped me cope with situations that were out of my control. It seemed to help me, at least for the moment, forget about the anger that was deep down inside of me.

One day a friend of mine asked me if I wanted to stop. I said, "No!" I told him that it was something I needed in my life. That same friend continued to compassionately compel me to stop cutting myself. My cutting got more intense over time, and, in fact, one episode landed me in the hospital. I cut myself so deep, I cut an artery. During that hospital stay, my friend, along with an individual from his church, visited me. They lovingly told me of Someone who loved me and wanted to take all of my pain upon Himself. They explained to me the love of Jesus Christ. I knew that I needed help and could not continue down this road of destruction. They invited me to a program their church had on Friday nights. Later, I found this program to be Reformers Unanimous. During those Friday night meetings, I found Jesus Christ as my personal Savior and Friend. I have only been in the RU program for several months, but it has made a world of difference in my life. When I get the urge to cut myself now, I realize that I can go to my Savior, my Friend, and He will take that pain and anger I have deep inside and give me a calmness and peace like I've never had before.

What has helped me the most is the daily personal journal. Not only am I able to find God's message for me, but I am able to express myself to Him. In so doing, I now walk in a glorious freedom I had never experienced before.

Jamie's Testimony

I am nineteen years old, and I have just finished my first year of Bible College. I do not have a crummy or dysfunctional family. My parents are wonderful Christians. They love me unconditionally, and I love them the same. As far as my family and friends are concerned, I have it all together. But, you see, five years ago when I was fourteen, my boyfriend raped me. I am not sure if that is what made me start cutting myself, but it was not until after I was raped that I started cutting. One night, several weeks after that horrific event transpired, I was home alone. I was very upset and angry over what had transpired. I picked up a knife and started slicing my arms. I felt a relief like I had never felt before. I felt that I had found a way to control the pain I was experiencing. I liked the fact that I could control my life and feelings again. But, down deep in my heart I knew that this was not a proper avenue to take. It went against everything that I had been taught about God and His love for me.

Thankfully, the school I go to is associated with a Baptist Church that has a Reformers Unanimous Program on Friday nights. God so graciously intervened in my life as I walked into those doors at the RU meeting. There, I learned that I did not have to destroy myself any longer to gain some temporary relief. Through the second-talk counseling, I was able to unload my burden in a very vulnerable but healthy way. With the encouragement of others in my group and working through the RU curriculum, I no longer seek to hurt myself. I now only seek a deeper, abiding relationship with Jesus Christ. I have forgiven the one that committed such a horrific crime against me. I have forgiven myself, and I now walk in freedom with my Savior, Jesus Christ.

Joe's Testimony

My name is Joe, and I am in my mid-thirties. My story begins with a good upbringing in a good, Christian home. I came to know Jesus as my personal Savior when I was a young boy. I always enjoyed going to church and learning about the Bible. I had an uneventful teenage life. I graduated from high school and went to college and earned a degree in Economics. After college I had a rough time getting a job that I really liked. I ended up in a delivery job. It met my needs, and I was somewhat satisfied. However, I always felt like I was "jipped" into taking the delivery job. I was faithful to my church, and I eventually met a godly woman. We got married. Even though my wife and I both had jobs, we were having a hard time making ends meet. It always seemed that when our bills were paid, we either had no money left over or we were actually overdrawn. This stressed my life, and it also stressed our marriage. I eventually went back to night school to further my degree and land a job that would be more satisfying. This added even more stress, as the financial picture was the same and now I was gone more from the house. Our marriage was, again, having difficulties. Because I was trying to work as much as I could and go to school, I started to miss some of the church services.

Knowing that my wife and I were running into spiritual, financial, and marital problems, I started going to our church's Reformers Unanimous Program on Friday nights. I did not fully get involved. I was very hesitant and certainly not very committed. My wife had grown somewhat cold to the things of God, and she would not even entertain the thought of going to the RU program.

I finally finished my Master's Degree and became a Certified Public Accountant. I finally landed a job that I thought was going to be the answer to all of our problems. The job was quite stressful. Eight months into my job, I was let go. This was devastating! What I thought was the answer turned out to be just another part of the problem. My wife was so upset and started to talk about divorce. I felt that I was in a deep hole. So, one morning when I woke up, I felt that the hole was so deep there was no way out. Sitting there on my couch, I realized that the only way out was to commit suicide. My wife had gone shopping that morning with her mother so I was all alone. I went to the medicine cabinet and pulled two bottles of over-the-counter medications and took them all. About two minutes after I took all that medication, my friend called me. He said that God had placed me on his heart, and he was calling to see if there was anything he could do for me. I told him what I had just done. He immediately hung up, and within the next five or ten minutes, the police and paramedics were at my door. They came in and rushed me to the hospital where I received proper medical care that saved my life.

My pastor visited me that day in the hospital, and we discussed all the things that were transpiring. He told me that the answer that I was looking for was not in a job, financial stability, and not even in marital stability. He said my answer was only found in Jesus Christ. It was not like I didn't know that, but I just needed to hear it again. My pastor encouraged me to get back into the RU program. However, this time, fully committed! I have done just that. My wife is still non-committal, and I really don't know where our relationship is going. But, I do know where my relationship with Jesus Christ is going. I have a deeper, abiding relationship with Him more now than I ever had before. I can now say that regardless where anything else goes in my life, I do have peace and freedom with my Savior, Jesus Christ. I am so sorry that I attempted to take my life, but I am so thankful for the grace of God that has allowed me another opportunity to serve Him.

John, Jamie, and Joe could not take the internal pain any longer. They saw no way to escape their pain or sense of hopelessness except through continued self-harm and suicide attempts. Like John, Jamie, and Joe, many people of all ages and walks of life battle with the seemingly invincible problem of self-harm and suicide on a daily basis.

Does the scenario of John, Jamie, or Joe describe you or someone you love? Are you searching for answers? There are millions of people just like you or someone you know who are desperately seeking for their way out. Like John, Jamie, and Joe, many have found that way out. They were introduced to "the Way," the Lord Jesus Christ, and have joined thousands of addicts who have found freedom through this program called **Reformers Unanimous (RU)**. RU directs people to the Truth Who makes free. I speak of the Truth named the Lord Jesus Christ. Many have come to an RU meeting, facing a combination of destructive circumstances. Many have sought help on their own, like John, Jamie, and Joe, without any long-term success. Yet, these same people are transformed as they engage in the RU curriculum and participate in its extremely supportive weekly programs.

Thousands of these individuals are now productive members of society. Collectively, they are a living testimony that there is hope for you or for those whom you love.

Yes, self-harm and suicide CAN be eliminated from your life. There is hope! There is freedom! And, that is the gospel TRUTH!

CUTTING
THE TOPIC

Each individual that does self-harm or attempts suicide knows exactly how it makes them feel. They also recognize that the feeling it generates each time is fairly consistent. However, very few of them actually know why it makes them feel this way, much less how it happens.

As with addictive drugs, self-harm, and suicide attempts, it is amazing to learn how effective they are at masking the real root problem in a person's life. When someone is a cutter, like John and Jamie, their actions manipulate neurotransmitters in the brain that create a false sense of enjoyment and calmness. This sense of enjoyment and calmness is, of course, only temporary. As well, it is not reality. However, we have a very great Creator who made our body to secrete these neurotransmitters, and He has ways of doing so without the pain and misery of trying to harm ourselves.

NEUROTRANSMITTERS AND THEIR ROLES IN THE BODY

- Acetylcholine: stimulates muscles, aids in sleep cycle
- Norepinephrine: similar to adrenaline, increases heart rate; helps form memories
- GABA (gamma-aminobutyric acid): prevents anxiety
- Glutamate: aids in memory formation
- Serotonin: regulates mood and emotion
- Endorphin: necessary for pleasure and pain reduction
- Dopamine: motivation; pleasure

In this chapter, Dr. George Crabb, a board certified Internal Medicine physician and member of the American Society of Addiction Medicine, will explain to us the phenomenon and feeling behind the self-harm and suicide behavior that plagues many.

THE TOPIC: SELF-HARM

Can you imagine slicing your stomach with a razor blade or carving a design in your arm? How about burning your fingertips with a cigarette or scorching your palms with a lighter? Do you think you could ever intentionally break a finger, arm, foot, or a leg just because you wanted to? These are some of the activities behind self-harm. Most of the individuals that engage in self-harm behavior never thought they could do the above activities. But, now that they've started and experienced the calmness and sense of control from this behavior, they now find it hard to stop. In fact, they have become addicted to this self-harm behavior.

The testimonies of John and Jamie reflect some of the paradoxes of self-injury. They hate and like what they do. They want and don't want to stop. They cut, burn, and bruise themselves, but they do not want to kill themselves. They find shame and comfort in their scars.

Self-harm or self-injury is also known as "self-injurious behavior" (SIB). This includes such activity as self-mutilation, cutting, self-abuse, and para-suicidal behavior. For all practical purposes, self-harm is a widely-misunderstood phenomenon, characterized by repeated, deliberate, non-lethal harming of one's body. The greatest misunderstanding about self-harm is the assumption that self-injurers, like John and Jamie, want to die, and that their self-injurious behaviors are just failed attempts at suicide. This is not necessarily the case. I have found the best way to describe the reasons for self-injury, and they are as follows:

1. Self-injurers commonly report that they fill empty inside.
2. Self-injurers commonly report that they are under or over stimulated.
3. Self-injurers commonly report that they are unable to express their feelings.
4. Self-injurers commonly report that they are not understood by others.
5. Self-injurers commonly report that they are fearful to intimate relationships.

Self-injury is their way to cope with or relieve painful or hard to express feelings, and it is generally not a suicide attempt. In other words, self-injurers harm themselves in order to help themselves.

It is estimated that nearly one percent of the United States' population are self-injurers. Most are females like Jamie. As with John and Jamie, most self-injurers start harming themselves in their pre-teen or teenage years. Over fifty percent of self-injurers, like Jamie, were sexually abused. Many self-injurers deal with depression and severe anxiety disorders. Those that self-harm come in all shapes, sizes, and colors. Outward issues do not determine whether or not someone becomes a self-injurer. It has more to do with an inward inability to express feelings or cope with strong emotions. The primary reason people self-injure is to relieve emotional pain. It is an extreme, unhealthy, and ungodly coping mechanism that some people use to get through times of stress, anxiety, conflict, disappointment, failure, or heartache. Many self-injurers have never developed the ability to feel or express emotions in a healthy way. Self-injury provides relief, albeit temporary, from the pressure of pinned-up feelings. One individual in my office who was a self-injurer said to me, "I felt my emotional pain drain away with my blood. It is as though punching a hole in my skin deflated this balloon of intense, overwhelming feelings. The air of pain came out slowly, and the release only lasted a short time, but it gave me a much-needed release." This sense of release and euphoria comes from the same mechanism that cocaine and other drugs produce in the body. This is a temporary surge of the neurotransmitters in the brain. I have had other self-injurers tell me that they harm themselves in order to feel something or feel anything at all. They are numb emotionally. They have gone on to tell me that physical pain helps them acknowledge their emotional pain. Another described it this way: "It's like I was dead inside, and by cutting myself, it reminded me that I was still alive and could still feel something." Some self-injurers like Jamie, because of past events, are punishing themselves or expressing self-hatred. They don't want to die; they just want to blame, criticize, or punish themselves. This is not only true for those who have been abused sexually but also physically and emotionally. They replay imaginary video tapes of messages they heard from their abusers in their minds over and over again. Some of these statements they hear in their minds are:

- You are worthless.
- It is your fault.
- You deserve to be punished.
- You are bad.
- You have to pay.

In self-injurers' minds, cutting themselves serve two purposes: (1) It punishes them with pain, and (2) It allows some of their badness to seep out with their blood. It is a way for them to make up for their badness.

Self-injury can bring out a host of emotions, especially from people who do not understand the condition. These emotions can include:

- Shock
- Revulsion
- Anger
- Fear
- Disgust
- Shame
- Condemnation

Self-injurers have already felt these things about themselves, especially shame. Shame is what makes self-injurers wear long sleeves all summer long. They cover their scars and hide their injuries so nobody will know what they are doing. Shame is an incredibly strong, self-condemning emotion that keeps individuals, like John and Jamie, feeling badly about themselves and trapped in a cycle of self-destruction.

Self-injury is just as addictive as drugs, pornography, or tobacco. Remember, no one can make self-injurers stop hurting themselves. This is a choice that they can only make for themselves. However, it is a choice that they may need support to reach.

Another type of self-injury is eating disorders. These attempts at self-harm, whether starvation (Anorexia Nervosa), binging and purging (Bulimia), or extreme over-eating (Binge Eating Disorder), are covered in a separate subject book entitled, *Eating*.

I am often asked by a loved one, "How can I tell if my friend or loved one is self-injuring themselves?" The following are guidelines to help you evaluate the situation:

1. Does your friend or loved one have cuts or scars on their arms or legs?
2. Does your friend or loved one try to keep you from seeing their scars?
3. Does your friend or loved one wear long pants and long-sleeve shirts in hot weather?
4. Does your friend or loved one offer lame explanations for their injuries, i.e., "The cat scratched me."
5. Does your friend or loved one show signs of depression or anger?

If your friend or loved one answered **YES** to any of the above questions, it could indicate that they are engaging in self-harm behavior. Again, the above is not an exhaustive list, but it is information to help you evaluate the situation your friend or loved one may be in.

In closing this section on self-harm, just remember that all self-injury behaviors are silent cries for help.

THE TOPIC: SUICIDE

What is most troubling is that the suicide rate for people nineteen and under has increased in recent years. Adults may find these statistics shocking, but most young people are well aware of the problem.

Another troubling revelation in the Gallop Youth Survey's poll was the number of respondents who admitted that they have entertained notions of committing suicide. Some twenty-five percent of the respondents answered YES to this question, with seven percent admitting that they had at least taken initial steps to actually committing the act. It is estimated that one in 12,500 people between the ages of fifteen and nineteen can be expected to commit suicide. For children between the ages of ten and fourteen, the suicide rate is one in 100,000. This number may seem small, but it represents a huge problem. Boys are more likely to commit suicide than girls. It is my opinion that suicide is an emotional cancer of the soul. It truly is a silent crisis as Joe demonstrated in his life. This is a major dilemma for our churches, schools, and our nation. For the most part, the issue of suicide has remained unaddressed or inadequately responded to.

People find many reasons to take their own lives. Amongst the more frequent reasons why people attempt suicide are substance-abuse problems. Individuals having a difficult time coping with trouble at home, school, work, or finances (as was Joe's case), contemplate suicide much more than those who don't. Victims always show many warning signs.

Teenagers often have difficulty coping with life's challenges. In 1997, the Gallop Youth Survey published a "Teen Alienation Index." In that survey, twenty percent of the teenagers admitted to feeling confused, pressured, ignored, bored, afraid, angry, or tired. These teenagers also admitted to harboring thoughts of doing violence to themselves or others. Suicide is, of course, a problem that affects more than just teenagers. For people between the ages of twenty-five and thirty-four, suicide is the second-highest cause of death. For people between the ages of thirty-five and forty-four, it is the fourth highest cause of death. Overall, suicide is the eleventh highest cause of death in the United States.

It is estimated that every seventeen minutes, an American takes his or her own life. When a person does commit suicide, it devastates family, friends, and even their community. Just as awful is what may happen if the suicide attempt fails. Some people recover from their attempts to kill themselves, as was the case of Joe we read about earlier. But, what happens to the person who attempts suicide and fails and is forced to live with the wounds for the rest of his or her life? The damage caused by a failed suicide attempt may be physical as well as emotional. These individuals can be disabled with brain damage, confined to a wheelchair, or unable to work or enjoy a full life. According to the National Institute of Mental Health, as many as twenty-five unsuccessful suicide attempts are made for every attempt that is successful.

After the suicide attempt, one must face the reality of having made such a ghastly choice! This can be a daunting task. The suicide attempt of an individual can do more than traumatize the victim's family and friends. Sometimes, a whole community can feel the pain. There is a phenomenon called *suicide contagion*. According to the National Institute of Mental Health, one suicide can sometimes lead to another. In other words, the suicides could become contagious. Typically, suicide contagion occurs when the victim is exposed to a suicide committed by a friend or family member or through media reports of suicide.

One of the warning signs of someone potentially contemplating suicide, and a warning sign that Joe had in his life, was mood swings. Mood changes may not necessarily be toward sadness, though. People who were formerly quiet may become hyperactive. People who were friendly and outgoing may become withdrawn. Some people will become depressed, have trouble getting out of bed, not sleeping well at night, napping throughout the day, or waking up early in the morning and unable to return to sleep. Others may have changes in their appetites. They will begin to lose or gain weight rapidly. They may start to feel restless or uncomfortable around family and friends. Joe found it difficult to concentrate, and he started losing interest in hobbies and other activities that he once enjoyed. Others may start giving away their possessions preparing for their death. Older people, who prepare for suicide, may make out a will or make revisions to a will that already exists. Potential suicide victims may make a half-hearted attempt to kill themselves using a method they think will not work. Or, they may start taking risks with their lives, like driving recklessly. They may even start drinking alcohol and taking drugs. They can also lose interest in their personal appearance, and as in Joe's case, become preoccupied with death. Joe found himself entertaining thoughts that life was not worth living.

Research indicates that young people are often quite verbal with their intentions when they are contemplating suicide. They may make the following statements:

1. I would be better off dead!
2. Nothing matters, it is no use.

Who is at risk for suicide? Suicide among young people is a problem that is growing at an alarming rate. However, it is the elderly, particularly older, white males, who are most likely to commit suicide. Among white males sixty-five and older, risk goes up with age. Males eighty-five and older have a suicide rate that is six times that of the overall national rate. However, statistics indicate that anyone can fall prey to suicide. In fact, any young person can fall victim to suicide, i.e., straight-A students, athletes, gifted students, and the like. Students who struggle in school or students who simply seem to blend into the crowd are also at risk. But, there are many things that are common among suicide victims as illustrated in Joe's life. They experience strong feelings of stress, confusion, self-doubt, pressure to succeed, financial uncertainty, and other fears of the future. For teenagers, some may find the breakup of their parents' marriage too traumatic to face. Others may harbor deep feelings of stress over the remarriage of their parents and the formation of new families, in which they are forced to share a home with step parents or new siblings. Maybe the divorce forced them to move to a new community and enroll in a new school where they have no friends. Suicide offers a solution to these seemingly, insurmountable problems. One trend is the rise in suicide rates on college campuses. According to statistics compiled by the National Mental Health Association, suicide is the second-leading cause of death among people of college age. Some of the reasons for this trend among college students are obvious:

- College students find themselves away from home for the first time.
- College students are confronted with an unfamiliar environment.
- College students don't have their family and friends to rely on if they need help.
- College students generally find it hard to cope at college for the first time.

Another well-known fact is the relationship between alcohol and drug use in suicidal behavior. A review of suicides among young people between the ages of eighteen and twenty found that drinking alcohol was associated with higher youth suicide rates. In studies that examine risk factors among people that have completed suicide, drug and alcohol abuse occurs more frequently among young people compared to older persons. Alcohol and drug abuse lead many people down a road of hopelessness and despair. People consider suicide when they are hopeless and unable to see alternative solutions to their problems. Most suicide victims believe they have become a burden on others.

There is another strong association and that is suicide and eating disorders. Recent studies have demonstrated a link to suicide with eating disorders, specifically Bulimia Nervosa. Bulimia Nervosa is an eating disorder that primarily affects adolescent girls and young women. Individuals who suffer from Bulimia Nervosa stuff themselves with food (this is called binge eating or binging), then they force themselves to vomit or use laxatives (this is known as purging) to get rid of the food they just ate. Girls who suffer from Bulimia Nervosa have a morbid fear of getting fat. It is similar to the eating disorder known as Anorexia Nervosa in which girls starve themselves. In 1998, a poll taken by the Gallop Youth Survey found that ninety-two percent of the five-hundred teenagers questioned worry about what they weigh. There are many similarities among people who exhibit symptoms of Bulimia Nervosa and people who talk about suicide or try to kill themselves. Bulimia Nervosa is an addictive behavior much like drug or alcohol abuse. I have had many bulimics tell me that they find the cycles of binge eating and purging to be a way in which they relieve anxiety, which is the same way individuals seek release from cares through drugs. Many people who have survived their suicide attempts have reported feeling better about themselves as though the attempt to do physical harm helped them find a release from their tensions and anxieties.

Another issue that must be addressed in regards to suicide is the violence in the entertainment media. The first suicide depicted in a theatre was probably in 1595 when William Shakespeare's play, *Romeo and Juliet*, made its debut. The often-told and often-mimicked story is now quite familiar. Two teenagers defy their families by falling in love. When events and enemies conspire against them, their story ends in tragedy – they take their own lives! The progression of violence from that time until now has intensified greatly. During the past forty years, there have been more than one thousand studies on the effects of media violence. Most of them have drawn similar conclusions: VIOLENCE IN THE ENTERTAINMENT MEDIA LEADS TO REAL-WORLD VIOLENCE. In 1999, a report to the U.S. Senate Judiciary Committee contained these statistics:

1. The average teenager listens to 10,500 hours or rock music between the seventh and twelfth grades.
2. In a typical 18-hour day of television programming, a viewer can observe an average of five violent acts per hour.
3. One study of media violence focused on the programming available on ten channels and found 1,846 acts of violence depicted in a single day.
4. By age 18, the typical teenager will have seen 200,000 acts of violence on television, including 16,000 simulated murders.

The report did not just focus on television, but it cited the increasing reliance on violence in movies, music, and video games.

The 1999 Senate Judiciary Committee Report commented: *A preference for heavy metal music may be a significant marker for alienation, substance abuse, psychiatric disorders, suicide risk, sex-role stereotyping, and risk-taking behaviors during adolescence.*

The result of inundating young people with violent entertainment is quite obvious. They have become desensitized to violence, meaning they don't appreciate violent content for what it truly is. The Senate Judiciary Committee Report went on to report: *Having fed our children death and horror as entertainment, we should not be surprised by the outcome.* In 1977 when the Gallop Organization first asked teenagers between the ages of thirteen and seventeen whether they felt there was too much violence in the movies, forty-two percent agreed. A total of 502 American teenagers participated in that poll. In 1999, twenty-two years later, the Gallop Organization asked the same question of 502 teenagers. This time, twenty-three percent of the respondents said they thought movies were too violent. What happened during the twenty-two years in between? It's only obvious! Teenagers were inundated with thousands and thousands of hours of violence in the movies, television, music, and video games. Someone who grows up in a world where violence is common, they may not find stabbings, shootings, or poisonings in movies all that violent. Violence is to the entertainment world what nicotine is to cigarettes. The reason why the media has to pump more violence into us is because we have built up a tolerance. In order to get the same "high," we need ever-higher levels of violence. The television industry has gained its market share through an addictive and toxic ingredient.

NOTE: There is no question, though, that the one factor that attributes to most young adult suicides is drug abuse.

Approximately seven years ago, I was called down to the emergency room to help revive a seventeen year old who attempted suicide by hanging. The whole medical team worked feverishly for more than thirty minutes in an attempt to revive this young man. Sorry to say, we were unsuccessful. Toxicology reports found massive amounts of alcohol and opiates in his system. After this young man was pronounced dead, the medical personnel found this fragmented note in his jeans. It stated, "I just want to scream and cry. I can't understand why I feel this way, as if my life were cursed at birth. But, I know that I have failed at life, and it is so much easier to just drop out. Please try and understand that this is for the best. Life was just unbearable. Please forgive me mom and dad." The note was signed, "I love you, Mark."

It is estimated that in the United States, some eleven million teenagers under the age of eighteen have tasted alcohol and many drink regularly. Drugs are another matter. Despite the ongoing war on drugs such as marijuana, cocaine, heroin, and LSD, drugs still remain readily available in and around schools throughout the United States. Illegal drugs are only a part of the problem. Many teenagers have access to prescription medications in the possession of older family members or friends. Medications such as tranquilizers, pain killers, and sedatives often produce some degree of narcotic effect. Even non-prescription medications cannot be ruled out. One study found that sixty-four percent of young people who tried to take their own lives by overdose made the attempt by using over-the-counter medications, which are available in any pharmacy in America to anyone with the money to buy them. Studies have concluded that there is a definite link between substance abuse and suicide. A 1989 report on teenage suicide prepared by the U.S. Alcohol, Drug Abuse & Mental Health Administration stated, "Analysis of data for adolescents…document a close association between substance abuse and suicide." Young people who abuse drugs and alcohol were up to eight times more likely to kill themselves than teenagers who don't drink or take drugs.

You see, in many cases, depressed, stressed, or despondent young people turn to drugs and alcohol as a way of drowning their troubles. They hope that by taking a drink or getting high, they will find relief from their anxieties. Of course, this solution does not work! Once the drug or the drink wears off, all their troubles return. Meanwhile, the adolescent has added a new problem to his woes – ABUSE OF ALCOHOL AND DRUGS! Alcohol and drugs, without exception, make a bad problem worse.

As we know, suicide is an impulsive act, so drugs and alcohol will make a teenager act impulsively, thus, commit suicide. Some drugs are hallucinogens. LSD (known as acid) and PCP (angel dust) may cause their users to hallucinate and totally lose touch with reality while they are under the influence. In some cases, users of hallucinogenic drugs experience violent or suicidal feelings. Sometimes, young people start thinking about suicide because of their alcohol and drug problems. When they started using drugs and drinking alcohol, they were not suicidal or in any way depressed. They may have just been experimenting with the alcohol and drugs. Soon, they become alcoholics and drug addicts. Their lives cave in around them. They become alienated from their family and friends. They sink into deep fits of despair as they find themselves unable to shake their habits and straighten out their lives. In the meantime, their alcohol and drug addiction grows worse. Finally, feeling no way out, they turn to suicide.

There is no question that a stable home life can be a deterrent to suicide. Sadly, stability is often lacking in many American homes. Young people who learn they are capable of accomplishing great things through the power or God generally do not look for reasons to kill themselves. Getting young people involved in church and school are also deterrents to teen suicide. Many potential suicide victims feel alienated. They are loners who think no one cares about them. Oh, but Somebody does care about them! So, no matter where you may be in your contemplation of life, I want to share with you that there is hope. There is Someone that cares, and that someone is Jesus Christ!

All that John, Jamie, Joe, and the other millions of individuals in our society today are looking for is help to heal the hurt that lives down deep within them.

Friend, regardless of where you may be in your struggle with self-harm or attempted suicide, the good news is that there is life after self-harm and suicide. John, Jamie, and Joe found this life. For this to be accomplished in your life, there must be a change in your behavior. I want you to know that the only effective way of changing your behavior is changing the beliefs to which you hold. This will be the subject of the remainder of this book.

EATING

EATING
THE TESTIMONIES

Alexis' Testimony

My name is Alexis and I am from Iowa. I grew up in a good home with Christian parents who served the Lord. I was involved in our church choir, the Wednesday night children's program, and many other church activities. Some might say that I had the perfect upbringing because I was not subjected to drugs, alcohol, or any other harmful influences.

What brought me to Reformers Unanimous was five and a half years of suffering from anorexia. It had taken away all of my happiness and hurt those who loved me most. I began to study health magazines and compare myself to my two sisters who were both petite. I thought they were prettier than me. I thought that if I were very skinny, my friends and family would find me more attractive and love me more. I was wrong! I allowed Satan to tell me I was ugly, overweight, and anything but beautiful. My self image was distorted, because I had been blinded and could not see myself as others saw me. I could not clearly see how much my family and friends cared for and loved me. My addiction became so bad that I went from a healthy, 131 pound individual to a 98 pound unhealthy individual. At times, I would weigh less. I was hospitalized in an eating disorder unit for approximately one month. I tried secular treatment programs but felt they were a waste of time. I did not realize that there was a God who knew me better than I knew myself, and He wanted to enjoy a personal relationship with me. I found this relationship after coming to Reformers Unanimous. After attending the program for a month, I did not feel like I was "getting it." I was actually fearful that they might ask me not to come back. But, I am grateful that did not happen. It was shortly after that when God began to reveal Himself to me. I started listening to the Holy Spirit and yielding my meditations to Him. Friend, God has changed my whole life completely. He has allowed me to be given a second chance through His Reformers Unanimous Ministry. He has used it to help me blossom into a beautiful young lady.

One of the biggest blessings was becoming a member of the Joy Belles. The Joy Belles is a group of RU ladies who sing and share their testimonies with others. While on tour with the other ladies, the Lord worked in and through me. He broke me! He helped me stop listening to the lies that Satan was trying to tell me. The other members of the Joy Belles began to see small changes in me and could tell that I was looking to Jesus for help and direction. My life changed slowly everyday over the course of three months. During this Joy Belles' tour, I realized that my Savior reached His hand down to me, dusted me off, and was bringing out the new Alexis.

God is so good to me, and it is only because I have given my all to Him. I no longer want what I want. I only want what God has for me. He is the only One who can change me, and He is changing me. I want to praise God for the RU program, our church, and all the ladies who have become my friends and encouraged me. My personal walk with God has grown substantially, and I have a new strength in my life. I owe a lot of it to the "It's Personal" daily journal to which I am now addicted. The RU program's daily journal has strengthened my personal relationship with God like no other tool I ever used. My parents are so glad to have their daughter back! I can now see the "me" that God saw a long time ago when He chose me to be one of His very own. The beauty of the Lord is awesome! I love the new healthy weight I have gained. I love the new healthy person I have become with the help of the Lord. Now, when Satan knocks on my door, I let God answer it. I look forward to God using me in the future to honor, respect, and glorify His name.

Lindsay's Testimony

My mom started talking to me about being overweight when I was about seven years old. Only, she called it being "chunky." Even back then she warned me not to let myself get heavy or the boys would not like me. What she said made me feel different, like "Maybe I was not as good as the other girls my age." When my mom took me to buy clothes, she always had this funny look on her face that made me feel ashamed. I got the sense that somehow she was disappointed in the way I looked. I really wanted to please her, so I thought I could lose weight by cutting out deserts and carbohydrates, which were the things I liked best. My mom would always say that those things would just make me fatter. As a young girl, I figured my mom knew what she was talking about because she was always trying to lose weight herself. I tried so hard! I would throw away all of my candy. When I actually lost weight, the expression on my mom's face made me feel happy. Then, when I was eleven, my parents got divorced. That was the worst thing in my whole life. Shortly after my parents' divorce, when I was about twelve, my father gave me a workout video. He told me that he just happened to pick it up and that he thought I would like to see it. Down deep, I got the message loud and clear. That is when I really started working seriously on getting thin. After a while, I figured out the perfect way to lose weight. I ate less than I ever had before, and I started exercising a lot. I figured that I could please my dad and make my mom happier if I looked better. You understand? If I looked thinner! As I lost weight, my parents were like, "Wow! This is great! You are really taking care of yourself." So, I felt good about it even though I did not really enjoy getting up early in the morning and exercising several hours before school. As time went on, I had the food thing under control. I continued to eat less and less. Now, I was exercising not only before school but after school – almost three to four hours a day. As I looked into the mirror, it looked as though I was not getting thin enough. In order to lose more weight, I had to start going days without food. I had to invent all kind of excuses for why I was not eating, because my parents got upset when I did not eat at all. Then, I found this website about *pro-ana*(that's like being pro-anorexic). On this website you can find great tips on how to lose weight. My mom started to get on me more and more about losing weight. I thought to myself, "Go figure! One minute you are giving me all this grief about being chunky so I lose weight. Now, you are getting on me about being too thin. I can't please her!" Everyone that I hung around with kept telling me, "Stop losing weight. You are getting too skinny." But, all I had to do was look into the mirror and it proved to me that I was still fat. One day, while exercising in my basement, I passed out. My mother heard a crash, and she came downstairs to see what happened. She found me lying on the floor. She called 911, and they rushed me to the hospital where the physician found me severely dehydrated and malnourished. They actually told my mom that I might not live. I was in the hospital for six weeks receiving intravenous fluids and food. During that time, several counselors, social workers, and psychiatrists came by to discuss with me what they called an eating disorder. Some of the things they said made sense. I knew what was going on was not really making me happy. During the middle of my hospitalization, my aunt came and visited me. She started talking to me about my eating disorder, and I expressed to her the pain that I had deep down inside. I told her how I looked at myself. I told her how unhappy I was that I was not able to please my parents. I went on to tell her that I had to work harder for them to love me. My aunt, who is a Godly, compassionate woman, shared with me, for the first time, the wonderful love of Jesus Christ. She and I were able to talk for hours. In my hospital bed, I realized that Jesus Christ loved me for who I was. There I accepted Jesus Christ as my personal Savior.

I was eventually discharged from the hospital, following up with counseling. But, I started to attend church with my aunt. My aunt introduced me to a couple that was in charge of the Reformers Unanimous Program at her church. The couple lovingly embraced me, and in a sense, adopted me. I started to attend RU on Friday nights. It has now been several years, and I have been faithful to my Savior, my church, and the RU program. On a daily basis, as I spend time reading the Bible, meditating on the Bible, and praying, I have learned that no matter how I appear to others or myself, I am accepted and loved in the eyes of God. I thank RU for helping me come to this understanding of my position and my relationship with Jesus Christ. Alexis and Lindsay could not take the internal pain any longer. They saw no way to escape the pain or sense of hopelessness except through continued starvation. Like Alexis and Lindsay, many people of all ages and walks of life battle with the seemingly invincible problem of an eating disorder on a daily basis.

Does the scenario of Alexis and Lindsay describe you or someone you love? Are you searching for answers? There are millions of people just like you or someone you know who are desperately seeking for their way out. Like Alexis and Lindsay, many have found that way out. They were introduced to "the Way," the Lord Jesus Christ, and have joined thousands of addicts who have found freedom through this program called **Reformers Unanimous (RU)**. RU directs people to the Truth Who makes free. I speak of the Truth named the Lord Jesus Christ. Many have come to an RU meeting, facing a combination of destructive circumstances. Many have sought help on their own, like Alexis and Lindsay, without any long-term success. Yet, these same people are transformed as they engage in the RU curriculum and participate in its extremely supportive weekly programs.

Thousands of these individuals are now productive members of society. Collectively, they are a living testimony that there is hope for you or for those whom you love.

Yes, an eating disorder CAN be eliminated from your life. There is hope! There is freedom! And, that is the gospel TRUTH!

EATING
THE TOPIC

An individual who has an eating disorder knows exactly how not eating or, in some cases, eating and binging makes them feel. They also recognize that the feeling it generates each time is fairly consistent. However, very few actually know why it makes them feel this way, much less how it happens.

As with all other addictions, it is amazing to learn how effective they are at masking the real root problem in a person's life. The decision to abstain from food or the actual purging after food is ingested actually stimulates neurotransmitters in the brain that create a false sense of well being. This sense of pleasure and control is, of course, only temporary. As well, it is not reality. However, we have a very great Creator who made our body to secrete these neurotransmitters, and He has ways of doing so without the pain and misery of this destructive behavior known as eating disorders.

NEUROTRANSMITTERS AND THEIR ROLES IN THE BODY:

- Acetylcholine: stimulates muscles, aids in sleep cycle
- Norepinephrine: similar to adrenaline, increases heart rate; helps form memories
- GABA (gamma-aminobutyric acid): prevents anxiety
- Glutamate: aids in memory formation
- Serotonin: regulates mood and emotion
- Endorphin: necessary for pleasure and pain reduction
- Dopamine: motivation; pleasure

In this chapter, Dr. George Crabb, a board certified Internal Medicine physician and member of the American Society of Addiction Medicine, will explain to us the phenomenon and feeling wrapped up in eating disorders that affect so many.

Alexis and Lindsay, who we read about earlier, experienced the effects of having an eating disorder. An individual with an eating disorder feels as if they are trapped in an overweight body. To escape this feeling, she or he may go on radical diets and exercise regimes. Many people with eating disorders fail to recognize the seriousness of their disorder. They do not really see what the mirror tells them. A person with an eating disorder may resist help because they can not believe the truth others tell them.

REMEMBER: Maintaining a healthy weight is important; obsessing over every pound is not.

According to the National Institute of Mental Health, over half of individuals diagnosed with anorexia will eventually develop bulimia. It is estimated that eight million people in the United States have an eating disorder. Ninety percent of those with an eating disorder are women. Eating disorders usually start in the teens but can begin as early as the age of eight. Though eating disorders occur more often in women, men also suffer from trying to attain the media image of the perfect male body.

For most of us, when we look into the mirror, we pretty much see ourselves how we physically are – lumps, bumps, and all the like. You have a realistic picture of what your body looks like. You have a healthy view of your body image. Your body image is defined as the following:

1. How you perceive your physical appearance.
2. How you feel about your physical appearance.
3. How you feel about your body.
4. How you think others see you.

For people with anorexia and bulimia, like Alexis and Lindsay, perception of their body image is drastically inaccurate. They look into the mirror and see a seriously overweight individual when in truth, they are severely malnourished. We look at these individuals and feel that they are making these gross exaggerations to get attention or looking for some kind of reassurance. But, Alexis and Lindsay truly perceived themselves as overweight.

There are three major types of eating disorders:

1. Anorexia Nervosa
2. Bulimia Nervosa
3. Binge Eating

In this chapter we will look at each one individually.

ANOREXIA NERVOSA

Anorexia Nervosa or *anorexia* is deliberate starvation with the purpose of losing weight. Along with a lack of food, a person with anorexia can over-exercise and may use laxatives or diuretics to enhance weight loss. Alexis had a distorted image of her body, and the fear of becoming fat controlled her life. If Alexis would not have found the freedom from her bondage, her eating disorder could have led to physical and psychological damage and possibly death. Although anorexia can occur at any age, usually its onset takes place during puberty or young adulthood.

Many people only think of anorexia as the severe restriction of food, however, the disease is divided into two categories: (1) Restrictive Form and (2) Binge-Eating/Purging Form. The restrictive form of anorexia is the most common. Individuals with this type of anorexia severely limit the number of calories they consume and also engage in excessive exercise to lose weight. The binge-eating/ purging anorexic is when an individual eats during binges and then purges by using laxatives, diuretics, enemas, or self-induced vomiting.

Alexis and Lindsay exposed themselves to very serious and damaging physical and psychological effects because of their eating disorder. Lindsay was often very depressed and suffered from severe mood swings. With all anorexics, the lack of proper nutrition can damage the heart, liver, and kidneys. Anemia, swollen joints, and brittle bones also develop in individuals with anorexia. The idea and process of losing weight consumed the life of Alexis. In fact, after a while, she found it easier to withdraw from family and friends than to come up with more excuses why she was eating so little or not eating at all. She started having difficulty concentrating, and her school work suffered. Secrecy is a large part of being anorexic. Food and eating can become a well-planned ritual for the person with anorexia. Lindsay would sit down to meals with her family and very thoughtfully push the food around the plate, making it appear as if she had eaten something. People with anorexia can become obsessed with weighing, not only themselves but also every bit of food they consume. They meticulously calculate the amount of calories that lies in front of them. On the other hand, some refuse to eat in front of people.

BULIMIA NERVOSA

Individuals with **Bulimia Nervosa** or **bulimia** regularly eat large amounts of food in a short period of time, which is much more than an average person would eat in the same amount of time. In fact, they could eat and drink between 5,000 to 10,000 calories during a regular day. In most cases, the person with bulimia purges by using laxatives, diuretics, enemas, self-induced vomiting, or excessive exercise. Bulimia is the most common eating disorder. It is estimated that up to 4.2 percent of females in the United States will have a period of bulimia at some point during their lifetime. Bulimia, like anorexia, begins in adolescence. Those with bulimia have recurrent episodes of binge eating characterized by eating an excessive amount of food as noted above. They, then, have a compensatory behavior in order to prevent weight gain, such as self-induced vomiting, misuse of laxatives, diuretics, enemas, or other medications along with fasting or excessive exercise. Bulimic behavior is usually conducted in private not to arouse suspicion.

The individual struggling with bulimia will typically throw up after meals. They will run the water in the bathroom for long periods in the attempt to cover up the sound of vomiting. They will also engage in excessive exercise programs. You will also notice calluses or scars on the knuckles from forced vomiting. They will admittedly deny any type of eating disorder.

Like anorexia, bulimia is divided into two categories: (1) Purging and (2) Non-Purging. Purging bulimia is the most common form of bulimia. The person uses laxatives, diuretics, enemas, and self-induced vomiting to rid the body of calories consumed during the binging cycle. Non-purging bulimia is when the person uses other methods to compensate for binging behavior. Instead of self-induced vomiting or abusing laxatives or other forms of medication, the person with this type of bulimia may skip meals or over-exercise to rid the body of calories consumed during binging episodes.

As with anorexia, bulimia comes with its own set of complications such as fluid, electrolyte, and mineral imbalances, which can lead to dehydration and problems with the heart in regards to arrhythmias. Many of the physical complications of bulimia come from self-induced purging. These include the loss of tooth enamel, tooth decay, sore throat, kidney damage, esophageal tear, and stomach rupture. A common complaint that I see in my medical practice with those that are suffering from bulimia is a complaint of constant stomach pain and acid reflux symptoms. The abuse of laxatives may lead to dependence on them, which leads to rectal prolapse and hemorrhoids. As with anorexics, many bulimics suffer from severe mood swings and bouts of depression, which are further exacerbated by periods of isolation caused by the disease.

A very dangerous practice with many bulimics is their thought to use other drugs to increase their metabolism, and thus, purge calories. The most common drugs used by bulimics to increase their metabolism are alcohol, methamphetamine, and heroin. Perhaps the biggest complication of bulimia is the secrecy surrounding its practice. Unlike anorexia, in which the self-induced starvation becomes apparent, someone with bulimia can hide the condition for years. The purging, dieting, and exercising that occurs between binges helps the individual maintain a weight within or even slightly above the normal range. This allows the destructive behavior to continue for a lengthy period of time while the psychological and physical complications continue.

BINGE EATING

Approximately four million Americans suffer with *binge eating* disorder, also called compulsive overeating. Binge eating for them is not something that happens on special occasions. For them, binging is the norm. Binge eating is the most common eating disorder in America, even more so than anorexia and bulimia. These individuals with binge eating have recurrent episodes of overeating characterized by eating an excessive amount of food within a discrete period of time.

- They eat much more rapidly than normal, eating until feeling uncomfortably full.
- They eat large amounts of food while not feeling physically hungry.
- They eat alone because of embarrassment of their excessive food intake.
- They typically feel disgusted with themselves after eating.
- They have depression and guilt after they overeat.

Binge eating disorder can mirror bulimia except in one important way: Individuals with binge eating disorder do not purge their bodies of the food. It is felt that binge eating disorder is the most common among men and most common among adults. For the individuals that I have treated with a binge eating disorder, they say that feelings of anger, sadness, boredom, and worry could send them into a binge eating episode.

Along with all other eating disorders, binge eating disorder comes with its own set of complications. The one that is most obvious is related to excessive weight. However, not all individuals with a binge eating disorder are overweight or obese but most are. This type of eating disorder can lead to:

- Type II Diabetes
- High Blood Pressure
- High Cholesterol
- Gallbladder Disease
- Heart Disease
- Musculoskeletal Disorders
- Certain Cancers

Individuals with a binge eating disorder report more health problems, more stress, more sleep disorders, and more suicidal thoughts than do individuals without any type of an eating disorder. For many, feelings of self hatred and discuss fill their thoughts. Feelings of shame can drive these people with binge eating disorders to a life of isolation just like anorexia and bulimia.

All eating disorders are serious! It is estimated that without finding freedom from this bondage, twenty percent of individuals with an eating disorder will die. With the devastation that can occur with these eating disorders, the question is, why? With any addiction, why do these individuals continue in this destructive behavior? For most individuals that I have counseled, as well as with Alexis and Lindsay, they had feelings of helplessness and a fear of becoming fat. Alexia felt that the denial of food was a way to gain control over her life. They feel that they cannot control anything around them, but the one thing they can control is their food intake and weight. They often feel like eating is the only thing they can control. And, in a life that demands too much of them, they can decide how much food they can put into their mouths. Not eating makes them feel empowered as if they have gained some control of their lives. Ultimately, of course, this sense of control is destructive, and it traps them in a lifestyle that limits them physically, emotionally, and spiritually. Individuals with bulimia and those who binge eat consume large amounts of food to cope with stress and other issues such as rejection and loneliness.

Several years ago a fifteen year old girl was brought to my clinic by her mother who suspected that her daughter was bulimic. After talking with this young girl, she shared with me that she had been raped while walking home from school one day. After I completed my examination and evaluation, I felt that this young lady had *post-traumatic stress disorder*. She would intermittently experience flashbacks from this horrific trauma she had a year ago, and these flashbacks would trigger her episodes of purging. She told me, with tears in her eyes, that she felt a sense of relief when she purged. She went on to say that she had temporary escape from the thoughts that haunted her. She explained that when she was purging, that was all she could think about. She said purging was not very pleasant, but it was a relief from the terrible memories that plagued her. With her mother's permission, I did treat her medically, but, more importantly, I introduced her and her mother to one of my best friends who is a Reformers Unanimous director at our local church.

I also want to educate the reader in regards to a very destructive website known as "*pro- ana.*" The prefix "*pro*" means "in favor of" and "*ana*" is short for anorexia. The term "*pro-mia*" means "in favor of bulimia." The *pro-ana* community encourages individuals to continue in their eating disorder. The *pro-ana* website can trigger dangerous thoughts and emotions in individuals who have eating disorders or who are recovering from one. There is definitely a darker side to these websites. *Ana* is not anorexia, the life-controlling eating disorder, but it represents a goddess who promises a thin, fulfilled life in exchange for devotion to her alone.

The following are examples of statements from a *pro-ana* site:

1. Should I be in such a weakened state that I should cave?
2. I will feel guilty and punish myself accordingly for I have failed her (ana).
3. I must be thin and remain thin if I wish to be loved.
4. I must weight myself every morning and keep that number in my mind through out the remainder of my day.
5. You will always be fat and never as beautiful as they are.
6. Surely a calorie and weight chart will follow me all the days of my life, and I will dwell in the fear of the scales forever. (This is a mockery of Psalm 23:6.)

I am often asked, "How do you tell if someone has an eating disorder?" First, it is not unusual to be concerned about weight and appearance. However, if a friend or loved one has any of the following signs, it may indicate they have an eating disorder:

- They are obsessed with food, such as counting every calorie or fat gram eaten.
- They avoid foods that they once loved to consume.
- They exercise too much although thin and losing weight.
- They start to isolate themselves and become less sociable.
- They feel as though they are not good enough in anything.
- They never let you see what he or she is eating.

- They continue to lose weight even though very thin.
- They wear oversized clothes in an attempt to cover their thinness.
- They use diet pills or laxatives to lose weight.
- They throw up after eating (frequently goes to the restroom after eating).
- They experience depression and mood swings.
- They experience tooth loss and decay.
- They experience dizziness, dry skin, hyperactivity, fainting, yellowish tint to skin, and feeling cold all the time.

Of course, the above list is not an exhaustive list.

Most eating disorders stem from deep emotional, psychological, and spiritual roots. There are different ways of handling stressful events, but turning to anorexia, bulimia or binge eating should not be an option. The behaviors associated with an eating disorder make you feel like you are in control but the opposite is true. When you choose to give into the harmful behaviors of anorexia, bulimia, or binge eating, you are actually giving control of your life to your enemy, the devil.

The solution to your eating disorder is far more complex than simply eating balanced meals and keeping the food down. The problem will not go away and the bondage will not be broken until the root problem is dealt with. But, freedom is possible. Freedom does exist for you. You have tried everything you know to get better. You now see your desperate need for God. You have reached your breaking point, and you know there is nothing and no one else but God.

All Alexis, Lindsay, and the other millions of individuals in our society today are looking for is help to heal the hurt that lives down deep within them.

Friend, regardless of where you may be in your struggle with an eating disorder, the good news is that there is life after this kind of an addiction. Alexis found this life. For this to be accomplished in your life, there must be a change in your behavior. I want you to know that the only effective way of changing your behavior is changing the beliefs to which you hold. This will be the subject of the remainder of this book.

GAMBLING

GAMBLING
THE TESTIMONIES

Paul's Testimony

One of the biggest things I remember about my years of active gambling is the liar I had become. I can't remember all the lies I told when I was gambling. I lied about how much money I had lost, when I would be home, and where I was going. Everything was a lie! My biggest lie was trying to reassure my wife that I would quit gambling altogether after just one last time in the casinos. I did feel guilty about my lies, and I did realize that the worst of my lies were the ones I kept telling myself. My life of gambling, mixed with all of those lies, brought me misery beyond my expectations. I could almost literally smell the stench of my own devious soul.

My gambling began several years before. Strangely enough, in the beginning, I never wanted to go gambling. But, some of my friends talked me into going, and I reluctantly went. I enjoyed it very much, and I decided to play the slot machines again. I soon found myself going every night. It was love at first sight. I was addicted. All my life I had been responsible when it came to money, and over a course of a few short months, I did not have one dollar on me. In fact, I had twelve credit cards that were "maxed" WW out. I had used all my savings, and I had sold a lot of what I owned in order to be able to keep gambling a little longer. I usually would gamble far from work and home. I did not want anyone to see me. I remember coming home after a gambling episode and having to face my wife. She would just stare at me with eyes that told me she could not continue to watch me destroy our lives. I remember one early morning coming home and finding my wife waiting for me in the living room. As I looked into her face, she looked pitiful and defeated. I knew it was my fault. I felt so confused during this time of my life. Shame engulfed me. I had brought my family to poverty, I had no self respect, and I even contemplated suicide. There was a point in my life where I felt there was no hope.

It was one Sunday morning that my wife said to me, "Let's go to church." Our longtime friends went to a local church, and they had invited us to attend. My wife really wanted to go. I was trying to weasel out. It had been years since I had been involved in church activities. I had been worshipping at the altar of the casinos. During several periods in my life, I had been actively involved in church. I loved those times. But, even though those times were the cleanest and the best times in my life, I still was not ready to go back to church. My wife was relentless toward me that morning. So, I finally caved in and went. We loved the church, and we started going regularly. I started to find myself looking forward to Sundays.

The church had a Reformers Unanimous Program on Friday evenings, and my wife and I started to go. After we started to the attend RU, I found out that my needs, the spiritual ones, were getting met. I began to recover my soul. I felt great comfort in reading the Scriptures, and the people at RU were very friendly. The RU director was an excellent preacher and teacher, and he had a lot of energy. I began to get involved and sensed hope once again in my life. However, I figured that once the other people began to find out about my gambling addiction, they would think I was a hypocrite. So, I did not want anyone to get too close to me. All of a sudden, I was starting to have strong urges to gamble again.

All along, I had an intellectual understanding of God, but it had never made its way down into my heart as a personal relationship with Him. I had spent my life looking for happiness in all of the wrong places. During one Friday night service, I shared my heart with the others that were there. Instead of finding ridicule and rejection, I found tremendous love and acceptance from my brothers and sisters in Christ. The journey that I now have is one full of satisfaction and joy. God has allowed my wife and me to recover out of the many financial woes my gambling led us into. We faithfully tithe and give an offering, and we faithfully walk with him on a daily basis.

Paul could not take the internal pain any longer. He saw no way to escape the pain or sense of hopelessness except through continued gambling. Like Paul, many people of all ages and walks of life battle with the seemingly invincible problem of gambling addiction on a daily basis.

Does the scenario of Paul describe you or someone you love? Are you searching for answers? There are millions of people just like you or someone you know who are desperately seeking for their way out. Like Paul, many have found that way out. They were introduced to "the Way," the Lord Jesus Christ, and have joined thousands of addicts who have found freedom through this program called **Reformers Unanimous (RU)**.

RU directs people to the Truth Who makes free. I speak of the Truth named the Lord Jesus Christ. Many have come to an RU meeting, facing a combination of destructive circumstances. Many have sought help on their own, like Paul, without any long-term success. Yet, these same people are transformed as they engage in the RU curriculum and participate in its extremely supportive weekly programs.

Thousands of these individuals are now productive members of society. Collectively, they are a living testimony that there is hope for you or for those whom you love.

Yes, gambling CAN be eliminated from your life. There is hope! There is freedom! And, that is the gospel TRUTH!

GAMBLING
THE TOPIC

Each gambler user knows exactly how gambling makes them feel. They also recognize that the feeling it generates each time is fairly consistent. However, very few gamblers actually know why it makes them feel this way, much less how it happens.

As with all other addictive drugs, it is amazing to learn how effective gambling is at masking the real root problem in a person's life. Gambling actually manipulates neurotransmitters in the brain that create a false sense of well being. This sense of pleasure and calmness is, of course, only temporary. As well, it is not reality. However, we have a very great Creator who made our body to secrete these neurotransmitters, and He has ways of doing so without the pain and misery of the effects of gambling.

NEUROTRANSMITTERS AND THEIR ROLES IN THE BODY:

- Acetylcholine: stimulates muscles, aids in sleep cycle
- Norepinephrine: similar to adrenaline, increases heart rate; helps form memories
- GABA (gamma-aminobutyric acid): prevents anxiety
- Glutamate: aids in memory formation
- Serotonin: regulates mood and emotion
- Endorphin: necessary for pleasure and pain reduction
- Dopamine: motivation; pleasure

In this chapter, Dr. George Crabb, a board certified Internal Medicine physician and member of the American Society of Addiction Medicine, will explain to us the phenomenon, feeling, and ultimate destruction gambling has on an individual's life.

The world may call individual's with a gambling addiction "a compulsive gambler" or a "pathological gambler." These are words they use to describe the person who falls prey to this destructive behavior when gambling takes over their life. Gambling, however, is simply another addiction just like any other drug addiction or self-destructive behavior. All addictions have some common threads. They are:

- Craving or Compulsion
- Control Loss
- Consequences are bad, but they continue with their behavior.

All addictions involve a craving and compulsion to continue the activity, whether it is the taking of a substance or the repeating of a behavior such as gambling. Perhaps the hallmark of all addictions, including gambling, is the existence of a loss of control. All addictions involve a continuing of the behavior despite negative consequences. All addictions have negative consequences, but the addicted individual continues to practice the addiction even in the face of all the bad things that are occurring to them. Gambling addicts spend money they should not spend at all. They run up credit card debt. They spend all of their savings, and it does not detour their activity in the least. And, like all other addictions, not one gambling addict actually planned on becoming addicted. Many individuals that are addicted to gambling are also addicted to alcohol and tobacco. Again, I have yet to meet a gambling addict that planned on becoming addicted to gambling. They probably began like Paul and just gambled for pleasure. Then, they began to gamble to cope with depression or stress in life, and then it went into a full-blown addiction.

It has been established by the medical community that gambling increases the level of the brain neurotransmitter called dopamine that moderates pleasure sensations in the brain. Dopamine is an "upper." This is a feel-good chemical that is also activated in cocaine and many other drug addictions. Gambling also increases the level of endorphins, another neurotransmitter in the brain, which reduces the feeling of pain in the body and gives a sense of well being.

Many have asked me, "How does a gambler get to this dark place?" The answer is that it does not happen all at once. There are, in this specific addiction, certain stages that a person goes through.

FIRST STAGE: THE WINNING STAGE

This does not mean that they win something large in cash, but the sense or thrill of a potential win gives them that surge of dopamine and endorphins in their brain which reinforces this activity as a pleasurable one. During this time, the stress, anxiety, depression, or frustration that is associated with their life is temporarily replaced with this "good feeling" associated with gambling. Some also derive a sense of pleasure and well being by the environment that they find themselves in; one that is highly sociable and accepting, but one that is saturated with alcohol and tobacco. The addict begins to fantasize about winning the "big one." They want to become a "rich person."

SECOND STAGE: THE LOSING STAGE

As the addict continues, he will eventually lose at times. In fact, you end up losing more than you win! As they begin to lose, they sense this air of competitiveness, and for them, the gauntlet of gambling has been thrown down. The battle cry says, "I am going to win my money back!" The chase is on!

THIRD STAGE: THE CHASING STAGE

Paul was determined to win back all of the money he had ever lost. In order to do this, Paul started to bet more money. The increased amount that is bet and lost lends to more excitement. What happened in Paul's life and what happens in the vast majority of those that gamble is that they keep losing money. Paul found out that video poker and slot machines can induce a gambling addiction just as rapidly as one can become addicted to crack cocaine. These specific types of games are solitary games; a game between the person and the machine. The reinforcements are immediate, numerous, and intense. The repetitiveness of the slot machines and the potential to win on each roll kept Paul in a constant state of excitement. In his early days, he would take a small amount of money to the casinos and that would satisfy him. But, as time went on, he found that he needed larger amounts of money to ensure a "good" chance of recouping his loses, plus, he wanted to ensure that he could gamble for a longer time without running out of money. Paul was getting addicted to the "action," and staying in the "action" requires a larger sum of money. In this stage called "chasing," debt becomes a very real problem. Paul began to let certain bills slide in order to have money to gamble. He depleted his bank account, and he allowed his credit cards to get out of control. He found himself in a financial jam. At this time, he started to realize he did need some help, and this led him to the next stage.

FOURTH STAGE: THE BAILOUT STAGE

We now see Paul in a real jam; he is in a serious financial jam! Those addicted to gambling will bail out in different ways: (1) Some will borrow money from friends or relatives. (2) Some will mortgage their property. (3) Some will obtain more credit cards in the attempt to alleviate the problem temporarily. During this phase in Paul's life, he would promise to himself as well as to his wife that he would stop gambling. But, those promises never lasted. Paul obtained more and more credit cards. In a sense, he knew what he was doing to himself and his family from a financial standpoint, but he felt that his actions allowed him to keep gambling. This is what his addiction demanded. He was in a love affair with gambling, and at that time in his life, it was stronger than any other relationship he had.

Many individuals think that addiction to gambling is about money and trying to "get something for nothing" or "getting rich without working." They are wrong. The goal is not necessarily money. If someone addicted to gambling goes into a casino and hits a jackpot on the first roll of a slot machine, does that addict get up and leave with the winnings? Believe me, this rarely occurs. No, the addict will probably try to win more money. Addicts want to stay in the action. That is what they are addicted to. Action fills the gambler's basic need, and it allows them to escape reality, albeit temporary.

Even after a bailout or two, Paul continued to gamble, and his life continued to spiral downward. But, it is merely a matter of time before the world falls in around the gambler's head, because the laws of probability are always working against the gambler.

FIFTH STAGE: THE DESPERATION STAGE

In this stage, Paul began to realize that there was not a way out of the hole. His future looked hopeless. This is a horrible stage. This is a stage that many consider suicide. It has been estimated that two out of ten gambling addicts will attempt suicide, and one in ten spouses of addicts will also attempt suicide. Paul testified that his depression grew deeper and deeper, and he lost all hope of recouping his losses. On the other hand, he found out that when he would go gambling, it lifted his depression temporarily. So, he continued to gamble! He would gamble and lose, and then he would experience more depression, which only turned him on to more gambling. It truly is a "dog chasing its tail." Round and round Paul went as he spiraled downward, desperate to gamble. Some individuals will embezzle money or obtain it illegally. Paul started to sell some of his assets. Some female gamblers resort to prostitution while men steal or commit armed robbery. Too often gambling addicts surrender to their gambling addiction. They give up! They keep on gambling despite the crushing reality surrounding them. Their physical health deteriorates as does their mental and emotional health. One addict that I attempted to help in my medical office described this desperation stage as this: "Sure, I'll tell you what it is like to be a gambling addict in this stage. It is feeling the devil's breath on your neck as you sit there gambling until everything you have is gone."

People who suspect a gambling problem in themselves, a friend, or a family member may recognize the following warning signs:

- Increasing preoccupation with gambling
- Use of gambling as a way to escape problems or relieve depression
- Inability to stop playing regardless of winning or losing
- Lying to family members or others to hide the amount of gambling
- Impatience with family or friends
- Relying on others for money to relieve a financial problem that arose due to gambling
- Absenteeism and tardiness at work or school
- Neglect of responsibility
- Losing or jeopardizing an important relationship due to gambling
- Wide mood swings
- Belief when winning that it will not stop
- Gambling another day to win back money lost gambling

You can ask Paul or anyone else that has dealt with an addiction to gambling, and they will, without exception, describe a nightmare. All that Paul and the other millions of individuals in our society today are looking for is help to heal the hurt that lives down deep within them.

Friend, regardless of where you may be in your struggle with a gambling addiction, the good news is that there is life after gambling. Paul found this life. For this to be accomplished in your life, there must be a change in your behavior. I want you to know that the only effective way of changing your behavior is changing the beliefs to which you hold. This will be the subject of the remainder of this book.

HEROIN

HEROIN
THE TESTIMONIES

Sandy's Testimony

At the age of ten, I accepted Jesus Christ as my personal Savior in a church service in Akron, Ohio. I will never forget that day! You see, I did not grow up in a Christian home, and I only attended church sporadically. I did, at times, do some Bible reading, but, in general, I did not lead a Christian life. I basically was untaught, but I knew I was saved. My high school years were, to an extent, uneventful. After high school, I worked for a year on the campus of Kent State University. It was during that time that drinking beer and smoking marijuana were introduced into my life. Not long after that, a professor at Kent State University turned me and my friends on to LSD. That began a real change in my life! Eventually, a friend and I moved to New York City where we got caught up in the show-business world. I was introduced to many people who were ungodly, but the money and the drugs were very appealing to a young lady. After three years in New York, I moved to San Francisco. It was there I was introduced to heroin and cocaine. My "significant other" and I worked underground dealing marijuana. We supported ourselves for ten years. Because of our drug dealing, we had the best that money could buy. During this time that I was actively addicted, I gave birth to two children, a boy and a girl. During this time I was still heavily indulging in marijuana, nitrous oxide, cocaine, and heroin. I would stay up for days on end getting high and not eating. Needless to say, this was devastating to my health and well being. I used the heroin by either snorting or smoking it. I was always too fearful to use it intravenously. As my life began to spiral downward, and as I needed more and more drugs, my "significant other" and I became more desperate for money. Our friends were quickly deserting us. I remember several people over these drug years looking at me and saying, "What are you doing here? You don't belong here!" You see, as they looked into my life, they could see that something was different even though I could not see it myself. I remember one morning, as I was getting out of the shower, looking into the mirror and asking myself, "How will I ever get out of this?"

One day, some dear people from a local church knocked on my door. They, of course, did not know my desperate situation. We were being evicted from our apartment and would have to move in with friends or onto the streets. I was afraid of losing my children. These kind people, who knocked on a stranger's door, took time with me, showed me much compassion, and also prayed with me. After they left, I went into my bedroom, laid across the bed, and cried. I knew that God had something better for me and my children. Not long after that, I scrapped up enough money, and me and my children went to my father's house in Ohio. It was a rough trip. I was coming off "speed balls," and, at the same time, caring for my two children. But, God saw me home! My boyfriend and father of our children soon followed me. Eventually, we moved to Michigan. My boyfriend got a "real" job, and we finally got married. We were still partying, drinking, smoking pot, and whatever else came to mind to do. By this time, our third child was born. A family member that was in the area saw our desperate plight, and he invited us to his church. The church was hosting a pot-luck dinner, and we all attended.

When I walked into the doors of that church, all I could think was, "Where have I been?" I cried through the whole service. I could not even bring myself to shake the pastor's hand because I felt so dirty and convicted. Because of the shame and guilt I felt, I did not go back. However, two years later, two ladies came to my door. These women were from the same church. They had no idea whose door they were knocking on, but it was mine. As I saw them through the window, I quickly kicked my pot tray under the couch and invited them in. I was, in a way, reintroduced to the Lord that day. I knew in my heart it was now or never. I did go back to church. I did make my public profession. I did get baptized. I am a faithful student of that church's addiction program called Reformers Unanimous.

Reformers Unanimous changed my life! The daily journal has opened my eyes to so many Spiritual truths. I have also pledged my life to becoming a faithful, door-to-door, soul winner. For, you see, there were two very important instances in my life when God sent, each time, two ladies to my door when I was in great need. God has been so good to me. My children are grown, responsible, sober adults. I am so thankful to God that He saw fit to deliver them from the pit of foolishness I was wallowing in. My husband has had a hard time over these past years. He has had an ongoing problem with alcohol. But, just this past year, he has become a faithful member, along with me, at Reformers Unanimous. I know that he has a long way to go, but he is on the right path. God is so good! He loved me in spite of my stupidity, faults, and my sin. He lifted me up out of the filth of this world and set me on the Solid Rock. I thank God for Reformers Unanimous. I thank God for my local church. I thank God for His Son, Jesus Christ. Jesus **NEVER** did forsake me, and my friend, He will **NEVER** forsake you either! Sandy could not take the internal torment any longer. She saw no way to escape the pain or sense of hopelessness except through continued use of heroin. Like Sandy, many people of all ages and walks of life battle with the seemingly invincible problem of heroin addiction on a daily basis.

Do the scenarios of Sandy describe you or someone you love? Are you searching for answers? There are millions of people just like you or someone you know who are desperately seeking for their way out. Like Sandy, many have found that way out. They were introduced to "the Way," the Lord Jesus Christ, and have joined thousands of addicts who have found freedom through this program called **Reformers Unanimous (RU)**. RU directs people to the Truth Who makes free. I speak of the Truth named the Lord Jesus Christ. Many have come to an RU meeting, facing a combination of destructive circumstances. Many have sought treatment, like Sandy, without any long-term success. Yet, these same people are transformed as they engage in the RU curriculum and participate in its extremely supportive weekly programs.

Thousands of these individuals are now productive members of society. Collectively, they are a living testimony that there is hope for you or for those whom you love.

Yes, heroin CAN be eliminated from your life. There is hope! There is freedom! And, that is the gospel TRUTH!

HEROIN
THE TOPIC

Each heroin user knows exactly how heroin makes them feel. They also recognize that the feeling it generates each time is fairly consistent. However, very few users actually know why it makes them feel this way, much less how it happens.

As with all other addictive drugs, it is amazing to learn how effective Heroin is at masking the real root problem in a person's life. Heroin actually stimulates neurotransmitters in the brain that create a false sense of enjoyment. This sense of pleasure is, of course, only temporal. As well, it is not reality. However, we have a very great Creator who made our body to secrete these neurotransmitters, and He has ways of doing so without the pain and misery of illegal and destructive habit forming drugs.

NEUROTRANSMITTERS AND THEIR ROLES IN THE BODY:

- Acetylcholine: stimulates muscles, aids in sleep cycle
- Norepinephrine: similar to adrenaline, increases heart rate; helps form memories
- GABA (gamma-aminobutyric acid): prevents anxiety
- Glutamate: aids in memory formation
- Serotonin: regulates mood and emotion
- Endorphin: necessary for pleasure and pain reduction
- Dopamine: motivation; pleasure

In this chapter, Dr. George Crabb, a board certified Internal Medicine physician and member of the American Society of Addiction Medicine, will explain to us the phenomenon and feeling of this mood and mind altering drug of choice for so many.

Sandy, who we read about in chapter two, experienced the effects that come from a resin that is found in the seed pod of the Asian poppy. Several different drugs that have been developed from this one, single source includes opium, morphine, codeine, and the topic of this book, HEROIN. Sandy fell into a large group of people that abuse heroin. In fact, heroin is the most commonly-abused opioid. The reason it is the most abused of that family is that it is one of the fastest acting opioid drugs. Sandy would get higher faster using heroin than any other opioid drug. Heroin is developed from morphine and is generally found as a brown or white powder.

Heroin that is sold on the street is rarely pure. While the most efficient method of using heroin is to inject it, the drug can also be smoked or sniffed. In fact, as the fear of communicable diseases, such as HIV, has grown from the sharing of needles, it is more popular today for the user to smoke or sniff the drug.

Sandy testified that she would have a euphoric feeling immediately after taking the heroin. To understand the effects of heroin on Sandy, we must first look at how it worked on her brain. The heroin interacts with the body's biological system. The chemical composition of heroin is such that there is a "key" that imitates the body's natural endorphins. As Sandy would use the heroin, it would be absorbed into her blood system and then cross her blood-brain barrier, saturating the brain tissue. There, it would be able to attach to endorphin receptors, taking the place of the naturally-occurring endorphins. Endorphin receptors are located in various parts of the brain, and this leads to the specific effects and consequences of the drug. One of the areas that has a high concentration of endorphin receptors is the area of the brain that controls pain. As the heroin attached itself to these receptors in Sandy's brain, they would make her feel less pain. Her surroundings would feel less threatening or dangerous, which can lead to risky behavior. There is also a calmness and a happiness that many users of heroin report. The euphoria that Sandy received, as well as the many other heroin addicts, is why so many individuals become addicted to heroin. Besides feeling this euphoria (calmness and happiness), the heroin, as it binds to other endorphin receptors in the brain and in the body, also has consequences. The user will have a decreased mental function. In a sense, they will feel as if they are in a cloud. Their actions are often diminished. Their breathing can slow down, and, in fact, may even shut down causing respiratory arrest. Sandy would complain of a dry mouth and a heavy feeling in all of her extremities coupled with occasional bouts of nausea, vomiting, and restlessness. Hunger and thirst are decreased, leading to dehydration and malnutrition. Along with the initial euphoria, there can also be significant mood swings, lethargy, and depression. The lifestyle that Sandy led, as well as all other heroin users, was one of a constant threat of disease and violence.

A common practice in this culture is to combine heroin with cocaine. This is a practice called "speed balling." Thus, combined with any side effects from the heroin, one must also deal with problems from the cocaine. This practice is more dangerous because drugs taken in combination can magnify not only the "high" but also their side effects. "Speed balling" is a deadly combination! This combination brings together a stimulant (cocaine) with the heroin to cancel the effects of the drugs. The cocaine keeps a user from falling asleep or succumbing to the lethargy that the heroin brings on, and the heroin helps control the hyper-activeness that occurs when cocaine is ingested.

There are many long-term effects of heroin addiction. Because heroin is commonly injected intravenously, many addicts' veins collapse. With most heroin users utilizing dirty needles to inject, they are at significant risk for infections in the right side of the heart as well as the valvular structures in the heart. This infection is called *endocarditis*. Communicable diseases such as HIV, hepatitis B, hepatitis C, and the like are more common in those that inject heroin. But, the most serious side effect of heroin use is the respiratory depression that it causes. This can occur with a single dose, but as a person continues in their addiction, tolerance occurs. This transpired in Sandy's life. She found herself having to take more and more of the drug to attempt to get a high. Respiratory depression (or the slowing down of the breathing rate) can be fatal, as the lungs and heart can slow down until they stop. I have personally witnessed, in my eighteen years of medical practice, several individuals that were brought into the emergency room with respiratory failure from heroin use. In spite of all the medical efforts, they could not be resuscitated. It is a common statement from their family and/or friends that they were continually escalating the amount of their heroin use.

Sandy would continue to let you know that during her active addiction to heroin that she would frequently be ill from colds or the flu. Heroin use suppresses the immune system, making the user more susceptible to infection. Heroin also disrupts the endocrine system. It can also lead to severe constipation, which can result in a bowel obstruction or a disease known as *paralytic ileus*, which is paralysis of the intestines.

There are not only consequences to the heroin drug itself but also to the additives it contains. The additives themselves can be poisonous. These additives are looked at as foreign chemicals to the body and can clog the blood stream, especially in the blood vessels leading to the lungs, brain, kidneys, heart, or other vital organs. This leads to permanent damage to the organs, which the user of heroin will suffer for the rest of their life. A very horrific aspect of heroin use, especially in those who inject the drug intravenously, is the high risk of communicable diseases, such as:

- Human Immunodeficiency Virus (HIV)
- Hepatitis A (HAV)
- Hepatitis B (HBV)
- Hepatitis C (HCV)

All of the above are severe viral infections that can ravage the body and even cause death.

A huge problem with heroin is the aspect of tolerance. Tolerance refers to the user's inability to achieve the desired high with the same dosage he or she started out with. Sandy experienced tolerance to heroin first hand. She would continually raise the doses of the heroin that she would take in order to feel like she did the first time she used it. However, she never achieved that "first high." Tolerance is dangerous! The more heroin that is put into the body, the greater the chances are of unwanted side effects and consequences. Overdose can also occur. Overdose is the worst possible consequence of heroin use. It is also, however, the most common. As noted, Sandy developed tolerance to the heroin quickly. This led her, again, to take higher and higher doses. Eventually, the addict will take a high enough dose that kills them. A high enough dose of heroin can suppress the respiratory or breathing rate until the individual stops breathing. This, then, leads to cardiac arrhythmias and finally death. While some overdoses are due to taking a lethal amount of heroin, others are caused by combining heroin with another drug, such as cocaine (otherwise known as "speed balling"). The chemical composition of heroin varies from batch to batch, so a user never knows how much heroin they are receiving in a single dose. Therefore, an amount that barely gave someone a high one day may be enough to kill them the next day. Although "speed balling" (heroin and cocaine together) receives more press, the most common deadly interaction is heroin and alcohol. You see, both are sedating drugs to the respiratory system, therefore, enhancing respiratory failure, cardiac arrhythmia, and death.

There are dangers of maternal heroin use. Sandy is now aware of the significant risk she placed her unborn children in as she continued with her heroin use during her pregnancies. The unborn child of a mother addicted to heroin faces an array of potential dangers before entering the world. Children born to a heroin-abusing mother deal with the following:

- Premature Deliveries
- Still Births
- Increased Risk of SIDS (Sudden Infant Death Syndrome)

An infant born to a mother addicted to heroin are born addicted themselves and go through withdrawal upon being born. These are known as "heroin babies." The withdrawal they go through is known as "Infant Abstinence Syndrome." I have stood at the side of a bassinet watching a 72-hour old baby start the withdrawal process from heroin. I remember standing over that precious little girl, innocent from any wrongdoing regarding drug addiction, begging God to have mercy on her life. This is another pivotal memory that has been seared into my mind that demonstrates the devastation of drug addiction not only on the addict but others also.

Heroin also causes biological changes in the brain of addicts. Because of these biological changes, heroin withdrawal is a very serious issue. Heroin withdrawal, to say the least, is depressing, debilitating, and, in some cases, deadly. As Sandy withdrew from heroin, she experienced muscle and bone pain. In fact, some heroin addicts have told me, as they went through the withdrawal process, that every aspect of their bodies would hurt. It is not uncommon for them to cry out that their "hair" hurts. Along with the significant pain that is associated with heroin withdrawal, they also become extremely restless. They also experience:

- Nausea
- Vomiting
- Diarrhea
- Chills
- Twitches (upper and lower extremities)
- Irritated Eyes; Eye Drainage
- Nose Drainage
- Extreme Anxiety
- Sweating
- Abdominal Cramps

While the symptoms of heroin withdrawal are more intense the first several days, they can last, in some degree, for several weeks. To say the least, withdrawal from heroin is severe! Sandy would describe to you in great detail that, without exception, her withdrawal from heroin was a nightmare.

Friend, regardless of where you may be at this time in your struggle with heroin addiction, the good news is that there is life after heroin! Sandy found this life!

For this to be accomplished in your life, there must be a change in your behavior. I want you to know that the only effective way of changing your behavior is changing the beliefs to which you hold. This will be the subject of the remainder of this book.

HUFFING

HUFFING
THE TESTIMONY

Lori's Testimony

I never thought it could happen to me – becoming addicted to inhalants! This was not a plan that I had. I had a pretty good childhood; going to church, playing sports in the community, and hanging out with my family. My mother and I were close, and we would hang out a lot together. My family lives in a small, Midwest town that is a very close-knit community. We always had things to do in the community as well as with our church.

When I was fourteen and entering into the ninth grade is when my life started to go downhill. Everyone looking at my life probably thought I had no problems. But, I had many problems. Although a lot of teenagers may feel as if they have problems, mine were rooted down deep in something that was not my fault – sexual abuse. You see, one weekend I went to visit my cousins. My uncle took advantage of me during that visit. He abused me! Dealing with something such as this is difficult, and trying to deal with it alone is virtually an impossible task. I felt at the time it was impossible to overcome. I started to look for ways of coping in my life; something to eliminate or deaden the pain I was feeling inside. I was offered help by my mom and dad, but I refused it at that time. I felt nothing at that time would help, until, I encountered drugs.

Now, it was my fifteenth birthday, and my friend offered me some marijuana. She knew what had happened to me by my uncle, and she said that the marijuana would help me. I tried it! It seemed that getting high was helping me forget my problems. However, without even noticing, I needed more drugs to get high. That is when I began huffing. I ended up inhaling almost anything I could get my hands on just so I could get high and have some form of sanity in my life. This went on for several years. My use grew and grew. My risk taking grew and grew. My actions landed me in the emergency room near death. I had almost suffocated as I was inhaling some chemical. Not enough oxygen had gotten to my brain, and I was brought to the emergency room by an ambulance. There in the emergency room, my wonderful parents were standing over my bed and praying to

God that He would help their daughter.

It was soon after that hospital stay that I, my parents, and my pastor had a meeting. It was there that our pastor introduced us to a program called Reformers Unanimous. My parents and I became actively involved in this Friday night program, where all of us have learned so much. I learned that the pain, anger, and hurt I had down deep inside was taken care of by Jesus Christ. I learned to accept His love and give Him my pain and hurt. In doing this, I walk in freedom now. I am healing on the inside. This program on Friday nights has truly made a big difference, not only in my life but in the lives of the whole family. I thank God for giving us the answer to our problems and that answer is JESUS CHRIST.

Lori could not take the internal pain any longer. She saw no way to escape the pain or sense of hopelessness except through continued use of inhalants and solvents. Like Lori, many people of all ages and walks of life battle with the seemingly invincible problem of inhalants and solvents addiction on a daily basis.

Does the scenario of Lori describe you or someone you love? Are you searching for answers? There are millions of people just like you or someone you know who are desperately seeking for their way out. Like Lori, many have found that way out. They were introduced to "the Way," the Lord Jesus Christ, and have joined thousands of addicts who have found freedom through this program called **Reformers Unanimous (RU).** RU directs people to the Truth Who makes free. I speak of the Truth named the Lord Jesus Christ. Many have come to an RU meeting, facing a combination of destructive circumstances. Many have sought help on their own, like Lori, without any long-term success. Yet, these same people are transformed as they engage in the RU curriculum and participate in its extremely supportive weekly programs.

Thousands of these individuals are now productive members of society. Collectively, they are a living testimony that there is hope for you or for those whom you love.

Yes, inhalants and solvents CAN be eliminated from your life. There is hope! There is freedom! And, that is the gospel TRUTH!

HUFFING
THE TOPIC

Each inhalant and solvent abuser knows exactly how huffing makes them feel. They also recognize that the feeling it generates each time is fairly consistent. However, very few "huffers" actually know why it makes them feel this way, much less how it happens.

As with all other addictive drugs, it is amazing to learn how effective they are at masking the real root problem in a person's life. Inhalants and solvents actually manipulate neurotransmitters in the brain that create a false sense of well being. This sense of pleasure and calmness is, of course, only temporary. As well, it is not reality. However, we have a very great Creator who made our body to secrete these neurotransmitters, and He has ways of doing so without the pain and misery of huffing.

NEUROTRANSMITTERS AND THEIR ROLES IN THE BODY:

- Acetylcholine: stimulates muscles, aids in sleep cycle
- Norepinephrine: similar to adrenaline, increases heart rate; helps form memories
- GABA (gamma-aminobutyric acid): prevents anxiety
- Glutamate: aids in memory formation
- Serotonin: regulates mood and emotion
- Endorphin: necessary for pleasure and pain reduction
- Dopamine: motivation; pleasure

In this chapter, Dr. George Crabb, a board certified Internal Medicine physician and member of the American Society of Addiction Medicine, will explain to us the phenomenon and feeling of this mood and mind-altering drug of choice for so many.

Lori, who we read about earlier, experienced the effects of inhalants and solvents. I am often asked, "What are inhalants?" Inhalants are any chemicals that are intentionally taken into the body for non-medical purposes by inhaling. Some of these products that inhalant abusers use are vegetable cooking spray, model glue, nail polish remover, canned whipped cream, and hair spray. All of these products contain inhalants, which are breathable, chemical vapors that can cause psycho-active effects. These are only a few of the products; there are many more.

Inhalants can be divided into four categories:

1. VOLATILE SOLVENTS

These are substances that vaporize at room temperature. These volatile substances can be further classified as industrial, household, or art and office supply solvents. Industrial or household solvents include such items as dry cleaning fluid, de-greaser, paint thinner, gasoline, and glue. Art and office supply solvents include correction fluid and felt-tip marker fluid.

2. AEROSOL SOLVENTS

Among aerosol inhalants are such items as spray paint, hairspray, deodorant spray, fabric protector spray, computer cleaning products, and cooking spray.

3. GAS SOLVENTS

These are gases used in household and commercial products or in the medical profession. Household and commercial products used as inhalants are butane lighters, propane tanks, whipping cream aerosols (whippets), and refrigerant gases. Medical gases include ether, chloroform, hyalophane, and nitrous oxide   (often called laughing gas).

4. NITRITE SOLVENTS

Substances in this category are not as well known and include amyl and butyl nitrites. Amyl nitrites (best known as "poppers" or "snappers"), when used recreationally, is a clear, yellow liquid sold in cloth-covered, sealed bulbs that make a snapping sound when broken. Butyl nitrites are sold in small bottles with such names as "locker room" or "rush."

While some effects of inhalant abuse are temporary, others are permanent. Hearing loss, for example, is irreversible. One of the scariest facts about inhalants is the age at which a person experiments with them. The average age of initial use is ten!

How inhalants are used is another question that is often posed to me. These substances enter the body when they are inhaled. The fumes are taken into the body by sniffing, which is inhaling the fumes from an open container. Secondly, fumes are taken into the body by huffing, which is inhaling the fumes from an inhalant-soaked cloth held to the abuser's face. A third way fumes are taken into the body is by bagging, which is inhaling the fumes from a paper or plastic bag that is either held over the face or pulled over the abuser's head.

In order to appreciate how dangerous these products are, as Lori found out, it is necessary to know how they affect the body when used incorrectly. Inhalants are very effective at creating a high. They work on the body very quickly, and effects can be felt as quickly as a few seconds. At the most, it might take a few minutes to achieve a high. Inhalants quickly pass through lung tissue and enter the blood stream. Once in the blood stream, the chemicals easily cross the blood brain barrier, a mechanism intended to keep harmful substances from passing from the blood to the brain.

Like alcohol, most inhalants are sedatives. Someone, like Lori, under their effects, can resemble a person who has had too much alcohol to drink. Many inhalants contain more than one chemical, and how that inhalant affects the body depends on how many chemicals it contains. Three common chemicals are toluene, floral carbons, and nitrous oxide. Allow me to briefly describe each one.

TOLUENE – Petroleum-based product found in wood, smoke, and emissions.

FLORALCARBON – A halocarbon in which fluorine has replaced one or more of the hydrogen atoms. Floralcarbons are used in many products, including anesthetics, refrigerants, propellants, lubricants, and water and stain repellents.

NITROUS OXIDE – This is most commonly known as laughing gas. Nitrous oxide is also known as dinitrogenoxide and dinitrogen monoxide. It is an approved food additive mostly used as a propellant in such canned products as whipped cream. It is also approved for use as an inert gas to replace oxygen in bags of snack products, such as potato chips. Nitrous oxide is also used in dentistry and in some minor surgeries as an anesthetic and for its pain-relieving qualities.

The above and other chemicals interact in the inhalants to affect the body in many ways.

The National Inhalant Prevention Coalition lists four stages in the development of symptoms related to solvent abuse. Lori experienced all four of these stages multiple times as she continued her inhalant abuse.

STAGE ONE: THE EXCITATORY STAGE – Symptoms that Lori felt during this stage were euphoria, excitement, exhilaration, dizziness, hallucinations, sneezing, coughing, excessive salivation, nausea, vomiting, and bizarre behavior.

STAGE TWO: THE EARLY CENTRAL NERVOUS SYSTEM DEPRESSION – During this phase, Lori would start to become confused and disoriented. She would have a sense of dullness to her senses, loss of self control, ringing or buzzing in her head, blurred vision, abdominal cramps, and insensitivity to pain.

STAGE THREE: THE MEDIUM CENTRAL NERVOUS SYSTEM DEPRESSION – At this stage, Lori became drowsy, uncoordinated, slurred speech, and had depressed reflexes.

STAGE FOUR: THE LATE CENTRAL NERVOUS SYSTEM DEPRESSION – At this stage, Lori became unconscious (this is what brought her to the emergency room). This unconscious state leads to very strange and bizarre dreams, seizure activity, and potential death.

With the dramatic effect that inhalants have on the brain, these chemicals were compared to cocaine in respect to brain damage. As might be expected, it was discovered that both groups (cocaine users and inhalant users) suffered from brain damage and compromised intellectual functioning. What came as a surprise to some was that inhalant abusers had more abnormalities and more serious brain damage. This was seen in the inhalant abuser's Magnetic Resonance Imaging (MRI) scans.

Inhalant abusers had greater difficulty successfully completing tasks that test memory and the ability to focus, plan, and solve problems than did the cocaine abusers.

If we think inhalant use only affects the brain, we are remiss. Lung damage can be caused by inhaling these chemicals. Inhaling spray paint and typewriter correction fluid can lead to liver damage. Kidney damage is a frequent result of using toluene-containing inhalants. Individuals

> **INHALANTS & SOLVENTS FACT**
> Inhalants are very effective at creating a high because they work on the body so quickly.

who sniff gasoline or other products that contain benzene are more prone to developing blood disorders such as leukemia and severe forms of anemia (the shutting down of the bone marrow). The muscles are affected by long-term inhalant abuse. One muscle in particular, the heart, plays a significant role in one of the most serious side effects of inhalant abuse.

During my medical residency in the Detroit area, I was introduced to the Jones family. I was called down to the ER in order to help revive a fourteen year old boy who was found in his bedroom with a straw from a can of computer cleaner still in his mouth. We did our best, medically speaking, to revive this young boy, but we had no success. After consoling the family, the mother shared with us that she had overheard her son and one of his friends talking about inhaling, but she did not think they were serious. So, you see, some side effects of inhalant abuse are deadly. What happened in this young man's life is called "sudden sniffing death." This is one, short-term side effect that many who participate in sniffing, huffing, or bagging activities have no idea can happen. And, it can happen the very first time an individual abuses inhalants. Sudden sniffing death usually occurs after a session of prolonged sniffing. Also, after a while, the inhalants can cause the heart rhythm to become irregular and beat too quickly, causing the individual to go into heart failure and possibly die.

Other short-term side effects of inhalant abuse, some of which Lori had, include the following:

- Slurred Speech
- Relaxation
- Euphoria
- Nausea
- Vomiting
- Dizziness
- Blackouts
- Death

Besides the above, individuals can die from suffocating on plastic bags used for huffing or bagging. They can die from inhaling their own vomit also. Long-term or chronic use of inhalants can cause tolerance. When this occurs, the user finds that it takes increasingly more amounts of inhalants to achieve the same results. So, individuals abusing inhalants must change the way the substance enters their body. For example, Lori, in the beginning, reached an acceptable high by sniffing. But, after a while, she did not receive that same high by sniffing, so she changed her substance or she went to bagging, a method in which the inhalant is taken into the body in a more concentrated, stronger form.

But, not all of the side effects of inhalant abuse are physical. Psychological and behavioral side effects of inhalant abuse include:

- Impaired Judgment
- Mental Confusion
- Freight/Paranoia
- Hyperactivity
- Anxiety
- Acute Psychosis
- Increased Violence
- Aggressive Behavior

I am often asked by parents and loved ones about signs that someone might be abusing inhalants. I give them the following:

- Complaints of burning sensation on the tongue
- Dazed, dizzy, or drunk appearance
- Nausea and/or loss of appetite
- Development of peripheral neuropathy
- Decreased vision
- Severe cognitive impairment
- Seizure activity
- Nasal problems
- Eye irritation
- Signs of paint, correction fluid, or other chemical products in unusual places
- Slurred or disorientated speech
- Unusual behavior: anger, anxiety, irritability, excitability, or restlessness
- Unusual odor on the breath
- Chemical odor on clothing

The individual may also start using street names for the some of the inhalants, such as:

- Air Blast
- Amys
- Bolt
- Boppers
- Hardware
- High Ball
- Hippie Crack
- Huff
- Locker Room
- Moon Gas
- Poppers
- Snappers
- Spray
- Whippets

Inhalants found in an out-of-the-ordinary place is also a good sign that someone may be abusing inhalants.

In 2005, the Monitoring the Future (MTF) survey found that the use of inhalants was up particularly among eighth graders. The MTF survey found that 17.1 percent of eighth graders admitted to using inhalants at least once. The use of inhalants by eighth graders reflects one of the most alarming features of inhalant abuse. Inhalants are usually the first drugs abused by young people. As noted in the life of Lori, who started with marijuana, she quickly went to inhalants when she was fourteen. The average age of initial use of inhalants is ten, which is about eighteen months before the average person first tries cigarettes and four years before the average, initial use of narcotics.

Studies have also shown that those who begin using inhalants at a young age are more likely to have an addictive behavior with alcohol, illegal drugs, and prescription drugs over the course of their life.

You may ask, "Why inhalants?" Since there are so many substances available for abuse, why would someone choose to abuse inhalants? Some of the reasons adolescents give for abusing inhalants are as follows:

- **Experimentation**
- **Peer Pressure**
- **Cost Effectiveness**
- **Easy Availability**
- **Convenient Packaging (easily hidden in the pocket)**
- **Intoxication Feeling**

Of the above reasons mentioned, maybe the main reason inhalants are attractive to those inclined to using a substance is their availability. It is safe to say that almost every home in America contains some source of inhalants or solvents.

Some experts call inhalation abusers a hidden population. Generally, individuals who abuse inhalants or solvents are not making drug deals on the street or buying and hiding drug paraphernalia (syringes, needles, or pipes). An inhalant abuser can just go to the kitchen cabinet and get what they need.

Because of this availability and simplicity of their intake, this abuse often goes undetected until the individual gets caught or decides on their own to kick the inhalant and solvent habit. When they decide to stop, inhalant withdrawal starts. When the body gets used to having a certain substance and the substance becomes unavailable, the body can object. In the case of inhalants, withdrawal symptoms can be as follows:

- Tremors
- Headaches
- Severe Nervousness
- Excessive Sweating
- Sleep Disturbance
- Severe Irritability
- Jitters
- Nausea and Vomiting
- Heart Rate Increase
- Hallucinations

Detoxification from inhalants does not take place overnight. Some of the toxins can remain in the body for a long time. Some can remain for a month or more.

When Lori described her withdrawal from inhalants, she described a nightmare!

All that Lori and the other millions of individuals in our society today are looking for is help to heal the hurt that lives down deep within them.

Friend, regardless of where you may be in your struggle with inhalant and solvent addiction, the good news is that there is life after inhalant and solvent abuse. Lori found this life. For this to be accomplished in your life, there must be a change in your behavior. I want you to know that the only effective way of changing your behavior is changing the beliefs to which you hold. This will be the subject of the remainder of this book.

METH

METH
THE TESTIMONIES

Cheryl's Testimony

Hello, my name is Cheryl. I was introduced to crystal methamphetamine at the age of sixteen. At my "sweet sixteen birthday party" my friend gave me as a present crystal meth. When I saw what she had given me, I was scared. I hesitated to take it but with pressure from my friend, I finally caved in. It did make me feel talkative and energetic. At first, I loved it! I then began to think of taking more. Through my friend, I was able to get more crystal meth. I was a little bit overweight when I was sixteen, and I found out that as I continued to indulge in crystal meth, it helped me lose weight. You see, before that, I hated how I looked, and I felt a depression hanging all over my life because of how I looked. But now, I was suddenly losing weight without even trying, and I thought that my depression had gone. But, then as I entered into my late teen years, my life started falling apart. I kept losing more and more weight. I remember looking into my mirror and could hardly believe it was me. I looked like a skeleton with thin, whispy hair. I had always prized myself regarding my beautiful teeth. But, as I continued to use methamphetamine, my teeth even began to rot away. Due to my physical appearance, I started hiding in my room for days at a time, afraid to come out because I was paranoid of being caught.

I felt that my mom and dad, and even the whole world, were after me. You see, everybody looking into my family thought things were okay. We lived in a nice suburban home, and my father had a respectable job. My father, however, was an alcoholic. My mother, although active in community affairs, was in a constant state of denial and depression. Looking at my family from the inside, it was in total disarray.

Soon after graduating from high school, I felt that my life was out of control. I tried to quit many times on my own, but, within a day, I was back at it. I don't necessarily come from a Christian background, but I found myself one night crashing off of the crystal meth on my knees begging God for help. Within a week of that prayer, as I was at a restaurant with a friend, on the table someone had left a piece of literature that dealt with Reformers Unanimous. I secretly grabbed the information and put it quickly into my purse so that my friend would not notice. Later that day, believing God had sent that to me, I looked at this tract, "Break the Chains of Addiction," and read it. On the back was an address where a Reformers Unanimous meeting was going to be held at 7:00 p.m. on a Friday night. I decided to go; knowing if I did not, I would end up dead. I went with great hesitation and fear, not knowing what reception I would receive. As I walked into the meeting, the group of people there met me with open arms of compassion. I knew that somehow they understood, and I felt that the answer for my pain was finally in front of me.

Now, I can tell you as I have accepted Jesus Christ as my Savior, and as I have worked the program of Reformers Unanimous and continue to do so, I have found a liberation in my life that I have never experienced before. Physically I have been restored, mentally I am content, and spiritually I am complete. I believe that I am a testimony that God is in the transformation business. God has changed my life! He has removed my desire for crystal meth and replaced it with a wonderful relationship with Him. I know that He loves me. I have finally found the Friend I have been looking for and that Friend is Jesus Christ.

Crystal's Testimony

Hello, my name is Crystal. I am a 27-year-old wife and mother with two children. As far back as I can remember, my life was always in turmoil. I grew up in a very abusive and alcoholic household. It seemed every night there were people getting drunk and then the fighting would start. My siblings and I knew that it wouldn't be long until we would all be standing outside in the cold, again, because mom was leaving dad - for good this time. We were tortured by this night after night, never knowing what was going to happen. I felt completely helpless. I simply wanted to run away as fast as I could. As I grew older, I buried those memories and did what I thought I needed to do in order to get through life.

While still a young teenager, I went to a close family member's house and was introduced to something that has forever changed my life. I was introduced to marijuana and allowed to drink. Oh, this was the life! I had finally found a cure to all my problems. I was definitely feeling no pain. Over the next several years, the drinking got heavier and the drugs got harder. I continuously needed more to get the same feeling, and I was always searching for the next level.

When I was seventeen, I met my husband, Bill. We were so much alike. He, too, had many bad memories that he was burying under a mountain of drugs and alcohol and that was fine with me. I mean, we weren't hurting anybody else. It was our life, and we wanted to live it our way.

Within three years, I had two beautiful children, Meagan and Savannah. We tried to slow down a little when the kids were born, but we needed to have some kind of fun, right? Besides, we enjoyed it....until one night in May of 2001. Bill and I sat down to get high and drink for a while, and he told me that he wasn't feeling very well. Then it happened. I watched my husband nearly die of a heart attack. He spent about a week in intensive care in a hospital in Pittsburgh. While he was there, I made up my mind that we were going to change our lives. For about a year we did; but as he got healthier, the "call of the wild" grew stronger, and we gave in.

For some reason, this time was different. My addiction absolutely took control of me. I didn't (couldn't) seem to think about anything except drugs. I stopped paying the bills. I started selling off personal items and furniture to make money. I stopped cooking, cleaning, and being a wife to my husband. Even worse, I stopped being a mother for my two daughters. This went on for about a and a half, and then it like I woke up. Only I woke up into a nightmare. My children were freezing cold and literally starving. We had been spending hundreds of dollars a day on drugs, yet we didn't have electricity. We had no water. We had no heat. We didn't even have food to feed our children. Where did everything go? Where is the car? What happened to my house? What have I done? I looked like a skeleton. My teeth were decaying and falling out. I looked like I had some kind of disease. My heart cried out, somebody help me!!! PLEASE!!!

All I could think of doing was going to the church where I went as a kid. I could remember my Sunday School teacher leading me to the Lord there when I was 8 years old. Many years had passed, but I knew that they would help. I began going to church on Sundays and to my surprise, so did my husband. Three weeks later, he got saved! AMEN! I thought that things were finally going to get better. Unfortunately, they just got worse. I tried so hard to do right, but I kept falling flat on my face. This happened again and again, no matter what. I had enough. I just wanted to die. I had failed as a mom and was left with no other choice. I called the pastor of that church and did the hardest thing I have ever done. I gave up my children because I could no longer take care of them. 's when I learned about Reformers Unanimous. AMEN!

Since attending RU, my life has turned around full circle. RU showed me that I was trying to change my life in my own power and has taught me how to rely only on Jesus Christ for strength. The Strongholds Discipleship Course has given me exactly what I needed from the Word of God for the things that I was about to face in my life.

However, the most effective tool that RU had to offer me was the *"It's Personal"* Daily Journal. It has helped me get right using the Bible in a way that has caused me to grow. It has also given me the accountability to my leaders that I needed. Through this program, I have become involved in my church and I have absolutely fallen in love with the Lord.

In addition to restoring my marriage, the Lord has given me the greatest gift. He gave me back my children, who by the way are both SAVED and serving the Lord, AMEN!!! I am so thankful that the Lord has used Reformers Unanimous to be that special something that God used to change my life.

(A note from Crystal's husband)

For years I was addicted to drugs right along with my wife. I stood by and watched helplessly as the devil used our sin to tear apart our lives. He stole everything from our home to my wife's beauty. If it was not for God using RU in her life, I would not have watched God restore life back into my wife. God not only gave her back her health, but He gave her back her beauty. You can see it every time you look into her eyes; and especially, every time you see her smile.

Cheryl and Crystal could not take the internal pain any longer. They both saw no way to escape the pain or sense of hopelessness except through continued use of methamphetamine. Like Cheryl and Crystal, many people of all ages and walks of life battle with the seemingly invincible problem of methamphetamine addiction on a daily basis.

Do the scenarios of Cheryl or Crystal describe you or someone you love? Are you searching for answers? There are millions of people just like you or someone you know who are desperately seeking for their way out. Like Cheryl and Crystal, many have found that way out. They were introduced to "the Way," the Lord Jesus Christ, and have joined thousands of addicts who have found freedom through this program called **Reformers Unanimous (RU)**. RU directs people to the Truth Who makes free. I speak of the Truth named the Lord Jesus Christ. Many have come to an RU meeting, facing a combination of destructive circumstances. Many have sought help on their own, like Cheryl or Crystal, without any long-term success. Yet, these same people are transformed as they engage in the RU curriculum and participate in its extremely supportive weekly programs.

Thousands of these individuals are now productive members of society. Collectively, they are a living testimony that there is hope for you or for those whom you love.

Yes, methamphetamine CAN be eliminated from your life. There is hope! There is freedom! And, that is the gospel TRUTH!

METH
THE TOPIC

Each methamphetamine user knows exactly how methamphetamine makes them feel. They also recognize that the feeling it generates each time is fairly consistent. However, very few users actually know why it makes them feel this way, much less how it happens.

As with all other addictive drugs, it is amazing to learn how effective they are at masking the real root problem in a person's life. Methamphetamine actually stimulates neurotransmitters in the brain that create a false sense of well being. This sense of pleasure is, of course, only temporary. As well, it is not reality. However, we have a very great Creator who made our body to secrete these neurotransmitters, and He has ways of doing so without the pain and misery of illegal and destructive habit-forming drugs.

NEUROTRANSMITTERS AND THEIR ROLES IN THE BODY:

- Acetylcholine: stimulates muscles, aids in sleep cycle
- Norepinephrine: similar to adrenaline, increases heart rate; helps form memories
- GABA (gamma-aminobutyric acid): prevents anxiety
- Glutamate: aids in memory formation
- Serotonin: regulates mood and emotion
- Endorphin: necessary for pleasure and pain reduction
- Dopamine: motivation; pleasure

In this chapter, Dr. George Crabb, a board certified Internal Medicine physician and member of the American Society of Addiction Medicine, will explain to us the phenomenon and feeling of this mood and mind-altering drug of choice for so many.

Cheryl and Crystal, who we read about earlier, experienced the effect of methamphetamine, which is a man-made substance that belongs to a class of drugs referred to as stimulants. These stimulants speed up the brain's activity, increase energy, and boost alertness. They give the user feelings of intense pleasure and extreme euphoria.

Cheryl used methamphetamine. This type of drug known as

methamphetamine powder is frequently cut or diluted with other substances and is snorted or taken orally. Crystal, on the other hand, used crystal methamphetamine, known as crystalline methamphetamine hydrochloride and also known as "ice" or "crystal meth." Crystal meth can be smoked or injected intravenously. Crystal meth will give a more intense high or rush than the methamphetamine powder form of the drug, because it is rapidly absorbed into the blood system. Crystal meth is more addictive than the powder form. What makes the crystal meth more addictive is that it is not cut or diluted, but it is generally pure drug, which is much more potent. Crystal would confirm to all of us that the high associated with crystal meth is longer lasting and more itnense than with either cocaine or methamphetamine powder.

Methamphetamine in both its crystalline and powder forms is by far the most addictive substance known to man. Both Crystal and Cheryl were quickly addicted to this devastating substance. In fact, the saying goes, "Almost nobody tries "ice" just once." In the medical field, I have run across a statistic that demonstrates that people who try crystal meth have a grater than 90 percent likelihood of becoming addicted to it within a year.

As Cheryl snorted the methamphetamine and as Crystal smoked and injected the crystal meth, the high they received was almost immediate. They both have testified and would testify again today that they had a sense of energy and alertness they had never experienced before. The drug, as it manipulated the neurotransmitters, dopamine and norepinephrine, in their brains, gave them a sense of competence, intelligence, power, and control that they had never experienced before. They felt hyperactive, and for both of them, they had an endurance that was never a part of their life. Also, as mentioned by Cheryl, she had almost a complete loss of appetite with subsequent weight loss, which is common among methamphetamine users. Cheryl would go for days without feeling tired or needing sleep. The euphoria associated with Cheryl and Crystal's highs came with delusions of power and a feeling of invincibility.

All of this "good feeling of methamphetamine" comes from the drugs manipulation of the neurotransmitters in our brain called dopamine and norepinephrine. After an intoxicating dose of methamphetamine, dopamine levels in the brain increase by 700 to 1200 percent. The brain is in a sense flooded with dopamine. Dopamine is the neurotransmitter used primarily in the mid brain. It deals with the personality, emotional, and motivational centers of the mid brain as well as the pleasure center of the brain.

So, as Cheryl and Crystal indulged in the use of methamphetamine, their brains became, in a sense, saturated with dopamine, thus, working on their personality, emotional, motivational, and pleasure centers of the brain. This, again, led to the elated moods and the artificial feelings of extreme happiness, which keeps people coming back for more of the drug.

Cheryl and Crystal, along with all methamphetamine users, generally go through a cycle when taking this drug. This cycle typically has several stages of predictable behavior, from extreme euphoria to severe depression. This cycle that Cheryl and Crystal lived many times is a part of the reason why they, as well as many others, become addicted to methamphetamine and why this drug can and will ruin countless lives. Immediately after Cheryl and Crystal took methamphetamine, whether it be in the form of crystal meth or methamphetamine powder, they felt a rush, a period that involved the most intense, exhilarated, euphoric feeling they had ever experienced. Along with this heightened sense of pleasure and arousal came an increase in their metabolisms, causing a rapid heart beat (tachycardia). This stage of the cycle is caused by the methamphetamine stimulating a surge of dopamine and norepinephrine, which makes the body hyper alert. The high which follows this initial stage of a "rush" lasts for several hours. In order to maintain this high, Cheryl and Crystal would often binge. This means that they would continue to take methamphetamine for several hours, although the rush they experienced is not as extreme as the first one because of tolerance. This binge stage can, at times, last for several hours to several days, depending on how long the addicted individual continues to take the drug.

Cheryl and Crystal would then experience what is called the "tweeking" stage. This is when they find themselves, after continued use of methamphetamine, no longer receiving the intense high they used to get. This stage is when the user becomes the most unstable emotionally, and there is a high probability for violence or other delusionally-driven activity. Cheryl and Crystal, during this stage, were unable to sense the euphoric effects of methamphetamine and became significantly depressed. Because of the negative effects of this stage called "tweeking," Cheryl would often use alcohol, opiates, or other "downers" in the attempt to negate these effects and induce sleep. However, combining methamphetamine with alcohol, opiates, or other sedatives makes the "tweeking" phase even more dangerous, not only to the user but to family, friends, and even law enforcement.

The "tweeking" phase leads into the "crash" period. Because Crystal had been using methamphetamine for days, she had little or no sleep, and in all practical purposes, her brain had become depleted of several neurotransmitters, such as dopamine and norepinephrine. Crystal's body needed an incredible amount of sleep to recharge and stabilize the levels of her neurotransmitters. Crystal, on many occasions, would crash for up to three days, almost sleeping continuously.

Cheryl and Crystal both suffered from the short-term effects of their methamphetamine use, which includes headaches and blurred vision. Cheryl had significant hot flashes, dizzy spells, dry mouth, tremors, and insomnia. Crystal, at times, would have her temperature rise to dangerously high levels. These elevated temperatures, known as hyperthermia, can lead to seizure activity, which, then, can result in death. Both Cheryl and Crystal had profound behavioral changes as they felt themselves coming off their methamphetamine. They would become nervous and irritable. They would become more confused and aggressive. After they crashed from their highs, both suffered from significant depression, which would only facilitate their craving for more methamphetamine. Cheryl had a common behavioral change frequently reported in methamphetamine users known as "picking." She would pick at the skin of her face and hands, causing scarring over time. This picking is a reaction to the sensation that bugs are crawling on the skin. This condition is known as formication. Along with these behavioral changes comes paranoia as well as visual and auditory hallucinations.

One thing that the methamphetamine dealer does not tell his customers is that methamphetamine is neuro-toxic to the cells in the pleasure center (nucleus accumbens) of the brain, as well as many other brain centers. This means that permanent brain damage can occur from methamphetamine use. One of my patients that was "recreationally" using methamphetamine told me, "Well, brain damage happens over a long period of methamphetamine use." I tried to educate this young lady that severe brain damage can occur after relatively light use of methamphetamine. I have seen many that have used methamphetamine in the past become crippled with memory loss, trouble with movement disorders, and learning impediments. Other individuals I have seen have had heart failure and suffered strokes because of the intense stimulation to the cardiovascular system of the body. Methamphetamine dramatically increases blood pressure, thus, potentially damaging brain, heart, and kidney tissue.

Crystal, in her testimony, tells us about the tooth decay that is common in methamphetamine users. They call it "meth mouth." It is a combination of tooth grinding, decreased saliva (secondary to the drug), and decreased personal hygiene and oral care because everything takes second place to the drug.

As you read the incredible effect that methamphetamine has on people's lives, including Cheryl and Crystal, let me share with you an individual I ran across in September 2007. His name was Donald, and he was admitted to my Internal Medicine service through the emergency room. He was hospitalized for a condition called "meth-induced psychosis." He presented to the hospital with erratic, irrational, and violent behavior. As I interviewed him the following day in the hospital room, I found that he was a 37 year old individual who had been addicted to crystal meth for several years. I found that before his addiction he was successful in the business world and had actually obtained a doctorate degree in economics from a local university. Since he met crystal meth, his life took a downward course. He had been hospitalized several times for meth-induced psychosis as well as for deep depression. As I looked at this 37 year old man, his skin was covered with abscesses from injecting the drug. He told me that he felt that he lived in a dark, shadowy underworld where he had no true friends and no one that really cared about anything but crystal meth. He told me that when he started to shoot up with methamphetamine, he thought he found the answer to his emotional issues. He was fired from his job when his boss found him one day injecting himself with methamphetamine. His family and friends abandoned him. He lost his home and cars and now resides in a dingy apartment with broken windows, sleeping in his clothes because he has no heat. He finds his days blur into one another, and between his highs, his moods plunge leaving him obsessed as to where he will find his next fix. Laying there in his hospital bed looking at me, he distinctly said, "I hate my life." My friends, I sat at the end of his hospital bed in sheer amazement. Here was a successful, educated young man that in just a few short years had been brought to nothing by this drug. I did what I could for him medically, attempting to optimize his medical condition. On two different occasions I spent time with him, attempting to guide him in regards to this destructive lifestyle and where he needed to go. I gave him information regarding the Reformers Unanimous Chapter at my church. As I left his room one evening after talking with him, I told him I would see him in the morning and that we would talk more. The next day I rounded at the hospital around 7:00 a.m. When I went to his room, he was gone. As I called to the nurse and asked where he was, she stated that the last time she had seen him was around 6:15 a.m. She indicated that he was sitting on his bed somewhat frustrated and appeared to be very anxious. We came to find out that sometime between 6:15 a.m. and 7:00 a.m. he had walked out of the hospital. To this date, I do not know where he is. This is not something fictional that is going on, but this is real life for so many people. Meth users can overdose. Obviously, the dosage is different from person to person, but any dose of methamphetamine is considered toxic. I have seen several individuals come into the ER with signs of an overdose. They come in with an extremely elevated fever, having repetitive seizures, tremors, and heart arrhythmias. We attempt to cool their body off with cooling blankets and chilled IV fluids. We also attempt to give medications to stabilize the seizure activities as well as medications to stabilize the heart rate. But, in too many cases, death is the end result. Many of the deaths that I have witnessed at the hands of methamphetamine are because the individual is using methamphetamine with other drugs, such as alcohol, heroin (hard balling), cocaine, and marijuana.

Women who use methamphetamine while pregnant or breast feeding put their child at risk as well as themselves. Methamphetamine use during pregnancy endangers the child and can result in miscarriages, premature birth, and low-birth weight. Permanent neurological damage can not only take place in the mother but also in the child. Methamphetamine will also be delivered to the baby through the mother's breast milk. The child is in essence taking the drug right along with mom with all of its consequences, including neurological damage and even death.

Withdrawal from methamphetamine is a difficult, dangerous, and potentially deadly process. Crystal suffered from severe depression, irritability, and extreme lethargy. Cheryl, on the other hand, also experienced the above but also had a tendency for violence and even had suicidal thoughts. These are quite common when an individual is withdrawing from methamphetamine, along with insomnia, shaking, nausea, sweating, and hyperventilation. Because methamphetamine is neuro-toxic, some consequences of their use may linger for a lifetime.

I am probably asked once or twice a month by concerned family members, "How can we identify if our loved one is taking methamphetamine?" I tell them that there are certain characteristics and behaviors that can be looked for if someone is using methamphetamine. The individual will:

- Speak quickly and incoherently
- Pupils dilated and eyes can be bloodshot
- Sweat more than usual
- Weight loss over short period of time
- Teeth will become stained
- Scabs and scars from tendency to pick
- Paranoia sets in
- Visual and auditory hallucinations
- Memory loss
- Depression
- Grinding of teeth
- Restless and tense

The above are indicators that your loved one may be using methamphetamine. All that Cheryl and Crystal were looking for was help to heal the hurt that lived deep within them.

Friend, regardless of where you may be in your struggle with methamphetamine addiction, the good news is that there is life after methamphetamine. Cheryl and Crystal have found this life. For this to be accomplished in your life, there must be a change in your behavior. I want you to know that the only effective way of changing your behavior is changing the beliefs to which you hold. This will be the subject of the remainder of this book.

NINE THINGS METHAMPHETAMINE DOES TO THE USER

1. METHAMPHETAMINE CAN MESS WITH YOUR HEAD.
  A. Delusional
  B. Paranoid Ideation
  C. Hallucinations
  D. Bizarre Behavior (can continue months after one stops using)

2. METHAMPHETAMINE CAN MESS WITH YOUR SOCIAL LIFE.
  A. Neglect Friends & Family

3. METHAMPHETAMINE CAN MESS WITH YOUR WEIGHT.
  A. Decreased Appetite
  B. Serious Weight Loss
  C. Sickly-Skeleton Appearance

4. METHAMPHETAMINE CAN MESS WITH YOUR MOUTH.
A. Loss of White Teeth
B. "Meth-Mouth" is Gross

5. METHAMPHETAMINE CAN MESS WITH YOUR NEIGHBORHOOD.
A. Make-Shift Meth Labs Can Be Set Up Anywhere
- Bedrooms
- Garages
- Children's Play Areas
- Motel Rooms

B. Serious Health Hazards To Everyone Around
C. Cooking Meth Produces Large Amounts of Toxic Waste
- Dumped in Yards, Alleys, and Streets

D. Meth Labs Can Explode
- Endangering Children
- Injury From Fire
- Physical & Sexual Abuse
- Overexposure to Toxic Chemicals
- Malnutrition
- Contaminates the Environment
- Lead Poisoning

6. METHAMPHETAMINE CAN MESS WITH YOUR MOODS.
A. Extreme Mood Changes
- Irritability
- Confusion
- Severe Depression
- Euphoria
- Anxiety
- Episodes of Violent and Aggressive Behavior

7. METHAMPHETAMINE CAN MESS WITH YOUR SLEEP.
A. Stimulates Central Nervous System
- Awake and Wired All Night
- Even Days After Using

B. After-effects When the Binge is Over
- Crash
- Severely Depressed
- Disorientated and Unable to Function

8. METHAMPHETAMINE CAN MESS WITH YOUR SKIN.
   A. Sores and Scabs Due to Constant Picking at the Skin
   B. Formication – Sense of Bugs Crawling on Skin

9. METHAMPHETAMINE CAN KILL YOU.
   A. Fatal Liver Problems
   B. Fatal Heart Problems
   C. Fatal Kidney Problems
   D. Fatal Stroke
   E. Suicide

PORN

PORN
THE TESTIMONY

Jeremy's Testimony

My name is Jeremy, and I am a 23 year old young man. I want to share with you how I found freedom from a 12 year addiction to pornography. At the age of 12, I had my first exposure to pornography. I was exposed to it by my so-called friends. What started out as something very innocent quickly became a crippling behavior that almost destroyed my life. After I was exposed to pornography, I was instantly hooked. I wanted to get my hands on it as soon as possible. I knew what I was doing was not proper. My parents raised me to know better. I was a straight "A" student all through school and well liked by all my peers and authority. I was a pretty good kid! I never got into much trouble and never did any drugs. I used all this as an excuse to indulge in my behavior. It dwelt in darkness like all destructive behavior does. I thought to myself, "Well, I am a pretty good person. What is wrong with a little indulgence into pornography? After all, it was not hurting anybody." This was a lie, and I bought it hook, line, and sinker.

All the while, my parents did not know what I was doing behind their backs. My destructive behavior stayed pretty well under the radar for most of my adolescent years. When I was a young boy, my father turned away from God due to some major trials in his life. When I was 17, my father got his life right with God. I remember the change in his life, and I was taken back by it. My father was my hero. I had never realized that he had been away from God. I thought of my father as one of the most upstanding men I knew. I also knew that he believed in God. The first time I remember God drawing me to Himself was when my father got his life right with God. Little did I know that over the next year God brought many people into my life that influenced me toward the things of God. My heart was being softened to show me my need for a Savior.

At the age of 18, my dad sat down with me and gave me the gospel message. I heard the gospel message many times throughout my whole life, but I never saw my need. I really did not understand it. I thought I was a Christian because my parents were. I remember when my father gave me the gospel message that night, I felt as if I was standing in a courtroom with "GUILTY" written all over me. For the first time in my life, I saw my need for a Savior. However, the one thought that kept coming to mind was, "If I accept Jesus Christ as my Savior, I cannot continue to indulge in pornography!" Part of me wanted to give it up and part of me wanted to hold on to my pornography. The truth was I liked it. What I did not realize was that Jesus Christ was the only One who could give me a new desire to do right.

In one ear I had the devil saying, "Put this off! You can make a decision for Christ later." In the other ear, I heard Jesus saying, "Come to me for salvation!" There was a great battle for my soul taking place. My dad could see that I was under deep conviction. He said, "If you see your need, you need to make a decision tonight. Do not put it off." I was glad he said that because it shut the devil up for the moment. I called out to Jesus that night and asked Him to save me. I truly believe that Jesus had lived a perfect life, died on the cross for my sin, and rose victorious over the grave on the third day. I knew there was nothing I could do to save myself. I understood that clearly, but what I did not understand was that Jesus was the only One who could give me a power to live a righteous life. The power to overcome pornography would never come from me but from the Lord.

When I accepted Jesus Christ as my Savior, I started to see pornography for what it was – SIN that God hated! I felt so much shame for my sin that I did not want to tell anyone that I had a problem with pornography. After all, I was the person who never did anything wrong, and I had a reputation to protect. I let my pride get in the way, and I truly believe that if I had sought out help from my parents or pastor during the first year of being saved, pornography would have never taken hold of my life like it did. I had a problem, but it did not completely take control of my life. I just assumed I could fight this battle on my own. That is exactly what I tried to do. I was actually able to walk away from pornography for a couple of months, but it was not too long until I indulged into it again. This began a pattern that would occur over the next several years.

It was at least a year before I said anything to my parents with what I was struggling with. Even when I told them, I was not completely up front with them as to the seriousness of my problem. Little by little they began to realize with horror just how big this problem had become in my life. My parents were shocked to learn how long this had been a part of my life. They were very involved parents, and they did everything in their power to see that I was protected from harm. The only thing that they did not realize was that we had a pipeline of filth being streamed into our home. My parents were naive to how easy internet pornography was to access. By the time I had come to my parents and pastor with my problem, it was already starting to spiral out of control. A lot of heartache could have been avoided had I just opened my mouth in those early days of being a Christian. The next few years would bring great pain to me and those who loved me. Even though I received counsel from my pastor and had tighter accountability from my parents, I found very little victory in my life. I could not go very long without messing up. I was continually up and down. One minute I wanted to serve God with all that was in me, and the next minute I was wallowing in pornography. Each time I looked at pornography, I would tell myself that I would not do it again and that this time would be the last time. My parents and pastor really did not know how to help me. I believed they felt as helpless as I did to fight this addiction. Every time I gave into pornography, it felt like cords binding me tighter and tighter. I felt the grip of the addiction taking hold of me and taking me much farther than I wanted to go.

What started as something very innocent at the age of 12 was now controlling my life and leading me down a path of great destruction. I found myself lying and being very deceitful in order to indulge and going into places I never thought I would go into. I remember looking into the mirror and thinking, "I am turning into a monster!" To the outside world, everything looked fine. Only those who were the closest to me knew of my struggle. In fact, I experienced great success in many areas in my life during that time. I graduated from college at the top of my class. I started a career as a graphic designer, which had been my dream job for a long time. In many ways, it looked as if I had everything going for me, but I felt that my life was truly falling apart. If there was not a drastic change in my life soon, I knew that everything I worked for would be lost. I was a functioning addict in every sense of the word, but I was ceasing to function. Slowly but surely every area of my life began to be affected. I felt like I was on a roller coaster that did not stop. I became very discouraged and wondered if I would ever be free from this addiction. What was sad was that I did not have anyone standing up to give me much hope. In fact, I was told by good, well-meaning people that I might not get victory in my life and that the Christian life was nothing more than a struggle this side of Heaven. They went on to say that my addiction was just something I would have to deal with, and eventually, with time, things might get better. I had a hard time accepting that! That was not what I found when I read the Bible. But, after about a million times falling, I, too, began to believe the lie that this was just the way it was going to be. I felt utterly and completely defeated!

I remember one day thinking that Heaven would be much better than the hell I was going through here on earth. I had no doubts of my salvation, but I was tired of living defeated. I also did not feel I deserved to live. I felt as if I was doing great harm to the cause of Christ and also to my family with the way my life was going. So, one day I chose to overdose on over-the-counter medication. After doing so, I realized that I did not want to die. I told my mom that I overdosed, and she immediately gave me something to induce vomiting. We did all of this on the way to the emergency room where I found out that my mom's quick action saved my life. I found out from the physician on call that I had indeed taken a lethal amount of medication. By God's mercy my life had been spared. One would think that experience alone would have been enough to turn me around. Not even two weeks later I fell hard. This time, it went to a whole new level. This was the fall that caused me to come to the end of myself.

Four months before all of this, my church started a Reformers Unanimous Program. Reformers Unanimous was the first place that I found hope for the first time. RU was the first place I saw real victory through Christ. I started going to the Friday night classes and began learning what a real walk with Jesus Christ is like. I was no stranger to reading my Bible. In fact, I was very disciplined in reading my Bible. I read it everyday; I read it on the days I fell. I thought if I read my Bible more and did more for God, He would surely give me favor and overcome my addiction. I was very faithful to church as well. I was told that one of the best ways to overcome sin was to just get plugged into church and work hard for God. Well, that worked on the days that I had something to do for the church, but the days that I was not in church, I messed up. I became church dependent. Really, I was trying to depend on my efforts. I thought that all of my service was my walk with God. Through RU, I began to see what a real walk with Christ could be like. But, after my last fall, I knew in my heart that God was leading me to make some drastic changes in my life. Finally, I was completely broken. I no longer trusted myself. I became completely open to whatever God wanted to do in my life. God opened my eyes to the fact that I had been trusting in myself for victory instead of Him. I had no problem accepting the fact that Christ did all the work for salvation, but I felt He expected me to be the one working at changing my life. The Lord opened my eyes to the fact that the same way I got saved was the same way I am supposed to live the Christian life – TOTAL DEPENDENCE ON JESUS CHRIST! This was a major revelation for me that completely changed my life. I soon came to find out that as I developed a dependency on Christ and as God became real to me through His Word, I no longer had an extreme desire to indulge in pornography. God made me free! I had never felt such freedom in my life. Also, during this time, God revealed to me the importance of obeying what He had shown me to be His will. Lack of surrender in the life of a Christian will always lead to failure and powerlessness over sin. When I became open to allowing Jesus to be the Lord of my life, I found what had once seemed impossible to obtain now became effortless in many ways. This was Christ doing the work in me rather than me trying to make it happen myself. The life of Christ in me became a reality for me. I began focusing on yielding to the internal persuasion of the Holy Spirit. God prepares me for my day in the morning, prompting me with Bible verses. As I meditate on the verses throughout the day, the Holy Spirit begins to lead me and guide me with the Word of God. I have begun a true walk with God and everything is changing.

I found out that pornography had been my most glaring sin in my life, but I also had many other areas in my life in which I was defeated. Worry was also a great stronghold for me, and God has begun to give me victory in this area also. The good news is not just that Jesus saves from hell but that He saves from sin – ALL SIN! Liberty that comes from walking in obedience to God's Spirit is absolutely amazing. I now work for RU, the ministry that pointed me to the only truth that makes free. I am enrolled in part-time Bible College and want to serve in the ministry for the rest of my life. I hope that Jesus Christ opens your eyes to the freedom that comes from a personal relationship with Him.

Jeremy could not take the internal pain any longer. He saw no way to escape the pain or sense of hopelessness except through continued use of pornography. Like Jeremy, many people of all ages and walks of life battle with the seemingly invincible problem of pornography addiction on a daily basis.

Does the scenario of Jeremy describe you or someone you love? Are you searching for answers? There are millions of people just like you or someone you know who are desperately seeking for their way out. Like Jeremy, many have found that way out. They were introduced to "the Way," the Lord Jesus Christ, and have joined thousands of addicts who have found freedom through this program called **Reformers Unanimous (RU)**. RU directs people to the Truth Who makes free. I speak of the Truth named the Lord Jesus Christ. Many have come to an RU meeting, facing a combination of destructive circumstances. Many have sought help on their own, like Jeremy, without any long-term success. Yet, these same people are transformed as they engage in the RU curriculum and participate in its extremely supportive weekly programs.

Thousands of these individuals are now productive members of society. Collectively, they are a living testimony that there is hope for you or for those whom you love.

Yes, pornography CAN be eliminated from your life. There is hope! There is freedom! And, that is the gospel TRUTH!

PORN
The Topic

For those who view pornography, they know exactly how pornography makes them feel. They also recognize that the feeling it generates each time is fairly consistent. However, very few who indulge in pornography actually knows why it makes them feel this way, much less how it happens.

As with all other addictive drugs, it is amazing to learn how effective they are at masking the real root problem in a person's life. Pornography actually manipulates neurotransmitters in the brain that create a false sense of well being. This sense of pleasure and calmness is, of course, only temporary. As well, it is not reality. However, we have a very great Creator who made our body to secrete these neurotransmitters, and He has ways of doing so without the pain and misery of indulging in pornography.

NEUROTRANSMITTERS AND THEIR ROLES IN THE BODY:

- Acetylcholine: stimulates muscles, aids in sleep cycle
- Norepinephrine: similar to adrenaline, increases heart rate; helps form memories
- GABA (gamma-aminobutyric acid): prevents anxiety
- Glutamate: aids in memory formation
- Serotonin: regulates mood and emotion
- Endorphin: necessary for pleasure and pain reduction
- Dopamine: motivation; pleasure

In this chapter, Dr. George Crabb, a board certified Internal Medicine physician and member of the American Society of Addiction Medicine, will explain to us the ramifications behind this behavior, which is a choice for so many.

Jeremy, who we read about earlier, experienced the effects of the destructive behavior of pornography addiction. To understand the effects of pornography on Jeremy, we shall first look at how it worked on his brain. Pornography has a powerful impact on the brain's function. Pornography stimulates a group of chemicals called neurotransmitters. Because of this stimulation, Jeremy enjoyed the effects of this elevation of neurotransmitters in his brain through experiences of euphoria.

Neurotransmitters are messengers between different nerve cells in the brain. Pornography, as it is viewed by the individual, increases the amounts of these neurotransmitters released in the brain (specifically dopamine), thus, exciting the nerve endings and sending out even more signals. The main neurotransmitter stimulated by pornography is dopamine. Dopamine is related to the reward system. Dopamine reinforces the feelings achieved during pleasurable experiences, such as laughing, eating, exercising, or work. Pornography directly activates these circuits and helps to essentially condition or stamp in behaviors that are not only necessary for survival but are highly destructive, such as pornography. Jeremy became involved with such destructive, compulsive, male-adaptive behavior because of the effect that the increased surge of dopamine in his brain had on him as a result of his pornography addiction. This led Jeremy, as well as many others, into a life of self destruction.

Pornography may well be the single most insidious element within this country, and the cause of a variable avalanche of problems including:

- **Child Molestation**
- **Incest**
- **Child Kidnapping**
- **Mutilations**
- **Murder**
- **Every Other Conceivable Type of Sexual Perversion**

Pornography is an addiction, and, like any other addiction, it will escalate. You cannot dabble in destructive behavior up to a certain point and then drop it. It continues to escalate until it destroys the person involved. Secular humanists tell us that pornography is no more than a harmless, albeit, colorful quest for pleasure. We are finding out differently, however. With pornography, as with all other addictions, sooner or later the appalling, final consequences will surface. Pornography is not without consequences! Recent studies in the medical community have demonstrated sinister results connected to pornography. Webster's Dictionary tells us that pornography is the *"depiction of erotic behavior as in pictures or writing intended to cause sexual excitement."* It involves such materials as books, photographs, television, movies, internet, and the like. All of the above depict erotic behavior and are intended to cause sexual excitement. In my medical opinion, pornography, like any other addiction, falls into **four categories**, and they are absolutely predictable.

1. ADDICTION

Pornography is as addictive as alcohol, drugs, or gambling. Pornography is not something an individual can pick up and lay down or escape at will. It takes but a short time before the individual becomes addicted. Sadly, a high percentage of printed pornography eventually falls into the hands of children.

2. ESCALATION

Addiction takes only a short time and then escalation sets in. "Old pornography" is not as stimulating as "new pornography." There is no thrill in going over what has been previously viewed. An individual hooked on pornography needs a steady diet of bigger and better thrills. How is this provided? It is provided by deeper and deeper excursions into greater and greater perversion. This is escalation. It is easy to picture how the process begins. Once the individual is hooked, he has to have ever-increasing "doses" of pornography, and these must be of a stronger and stronger stimulation to elicit the arousal originally brought about by previous pornography. What happens when pornography of any type is viewed? It has a specific medical effect on the individual. It has been demonstrated that an actual chemical reaction takes place in an individual's brain when he views any type of pornographic material. The chemical reaction mediated by serotonin, dopamine, and epinephrine causes these mental images to be imprinted indelibly upon the brain of the individual. They will subsequently be recalled with clarity and such force that the individual is unable to break the chain of events as he falls deeper and deeper under the influence of these unhealthy stimuli. These chemical reactions also have a resulting effect not only upon the mind but also on the body.

3. DESENSITIZATION

Once the individual indulges in pornography, bondage is sure to follow. He becomes addicted until it becomes something he cannot pick up or put down at will. At this point, it begins to escalate. He must now wallow deeper and deeper into perversion to satisfy the demands of a mind that is rapidly becoming warped by this disease of hell. Material that would have once been repulsive and horribly shocking now becomes acceptable and even commonplace. The man who would not have ever considered molesting a child now starts to "get his kicks" by watching child molestation (or child abuse) on movies or by reading about it. It no longer repulses him. He is almost another person. Incredibly, the hard-core addict can watch a woman being raped and have no normal reaction of revulsion. To the contrary, he becomes aroused and sexually excited by viewing this "ghoulish" scene. What has happened? He has become desensitized. Normal responses have been erased and moral and spiritual disintegration have set in until he is finally in total bondage.

4. THE ACTING OUT

We have addiction followed by escalation and desensitization, and, finally, the acting out of the role. After viewing films, reading such material, viewing it on the Internet, and gradually becoming more and more debased, the individual suddenly finds himself desirous of acting out the role he has been viewing or reading about. At this point, he may try to get his wife or girlfriend to act out the female role in such situations, whatever it may be. If he does not have a wife or girlfriend, prostitution is resorted to with strange women or even children against their wishes. The compulsion does inevitably develop, however, to act out the role.

Ask Jeremy or anyone else who has struggled with an addiction to pornography about the effects. They will, without exception, describe a nightmare.

Friend, regardless of where you may be in your struggle with pornography addiction, the good news is that there is life after pornography. Jeremy found this life. For this to be accomplished in your life, there must be a change in your behavior. I want you to know that the only effective way of changing your behavior is changing the beliefs to which you hold. This will be the subject of the remainder of this book.

Rx

Rx
The Testimonies

My name is Judy, and I am a twenty-five year old, single mother from North Carolina. I grew up in what I would call a typical American home. We attended church occasionally, and my concept of pleasing others and pleasing God was always based on my performance. I had a relatively uneventful junior high and high school education. I went to college and received my R.N. degree. Soon after college, I met a man that I thought I would spend the rest of my life with. We did get married and soon had a baby boy. But, soon after, he left for another woman. This left me all alone with a son less than a year old. The pain that I felt inside was unbearable. The loneliness was intense. I felt that the failure in our marriage was because of me. Over the next few years this pain, rejection, and loneliness began to build in my life.

A very good friend of mine invited me to their church one Sunday, and I attended desiring to find peace in my soul. Over the next few months, while attending that church, I did accept Jesus Christ as my personal Savior. Even though I was now saved, a child of God, and on my way to Heaven, the pain, loneliness, and rejection from my divorce still haunted me deep in my soul. I soon met another man at the church; a godly man who was very involved in the things of God. We ultimately got married. Everything seemed to be going wonderfully – a godly husband who took care of me and my son. We were involved in many church activities, but I was still haunted by that pain, loneliness, and rejection deep in my soul.

One day while I was at the hospital passing medications out to my patients, a patient of mine refused to take her pain medicine, which was called Vicoden.®™ As I went back to the medication dispensing area, I saw, still in my hand, that pain medication. Obviously, I was supposed to put it back into the proper drawer for future use by the patient, but at that moment I had a fleeting thought of what this medicine would make me feel like. Therefore, I went to the bathroom and took the Vicoden. About twenty to thirty minutes later, I felt a magical feeling. For the next several hours I literally forgot about that inward pain, loneliness, and rejection, which was something I was unable to do for several years. As the medicine wore off, my mind started to think, "How can I get more!" This was the beginning of a downward cycle of addiction to the prescription medicine called Vicoden.

Over the next several years, I would divert patients' medicines and use them myself. I also befriended several doctors in the hospital, and I would ask them to write me a prescription for Vicoden. I would tell them that I had a headache, I hurt my knee, or sprained my ankle. If I persisted enough, I would eventually get a prescription from one of them.

I started to drop off working with my husband at the church. I began to isolate myself from my husband and son, both of whom I loved very much. My usage got more and more intense. One day, while at work and after taking several Vicoden, my supervisor approached me. She told me that she thought I was acting somewhat different. I immediately rejected this accusation. But, I was forced to give a urine drug screen, which obviously showed positive for opiates. I was then confronted by my supervisor, and I came clean in front of her. Now that my addiction was exposed, my job was on the line. I feared what my family would think as well as my church family. My work demanded that I go to a secular in-patient program for two weeks in order to keep my job. I went and spent two weeks in that program. During the two weeks of separation from my family and church family, I had much time to reflect on what I had done and where I had taken my life.

During my in-patient stay, my pastor had visited on several different occasions. We started to discuss why I needed the help. I was able, finally, to discuss with him the pain, loneliness, and rejection that I felt deep in my soul from my previous divorce. I truly believe that was the starting of my healing process. That was the beginning of my walk of freedom in Christ. My pastor brought up that once I was released from the in-patient program, I should get involved in the Reformers Unanimous Program at our church. All during my addiction, I never really acknowledged that we had such a program at our church. When my pastor brought it up, it was like a light bulb going off in my mind. After leaving the in-patient program, I wholeheartedly jumped into the RU program. Through this program I have learned to give my pain, loneliness, and rejection to my wonderful Savior, Jesus Christ. I've learned that He loves me and accepts me no matter what. I can't tell you the immense freedom I now have in Jesus. I have worked through the RU curriculum, and I daily journal, which has been such a tremendous help in my life. Now, I can tell you that when I have any pain, loneliness, or rejection in my life, I don't turn to drugs. I turn to my wonderful Savior and Friend – JESUS! He takes that loneliness, pain, and rejection away and gives me that peace that is so satisfying. My husband, I, and our son are now back working in the ministry of our church and reaching out to the children in our community through the bus ministry. Also, we are reaching out to those addicted in our community through our local chapter of Reformers Unanimous. I want to thank God for giving me freedom!

Mark's Testimony

My story is not that intense or in-depth, but my story is still extremely destructive. I grew up in a great Christian home, attended Bible College, and entered a pastorate at a very young age. As I continued in my pastorate, at times I did not know how to handle the stress of that position. There would be many days that my life would be filled with anxiety, and many times I would have difficulty sleeping at night. As I was sharing this with one of my church members, they pulled out of their pocked a little blue pill, and they told me to take it at bedtime to help me sleep. Later that evening, having difficulty sleeping, I took the medicine. This prescription medicine was called Xanax.®™ It gave me a wonderful night's sleep and a calming effect the next day. I really liked the way it made me feel. Things did not bother me as much. After a few days, I did not have any more, and just in passing, I asked the church member if he had any more. He said he did, and he gave me a handful of Xanax. Over the next two weeks, I took those, and, thus, started my downward progression.

Knowing that I needed more, I went to my physician and explained to him that I had been on this medication for some time and that I would need a full prescription. He gave them to me. He did warn me about their potential abuse and the possibility of addiction. I told him that I was a minister and that it would not be a problem. I went on my way. I could not believe what I was doing. I was finding relief in a prescription medication. I knew this was not the answer, but I just could not pull myself away.

One Sunday night after the service, one of my dearest church members pulled me aside and said, "Pastor, I think you might have a problem." I can't tell you how that felt. At that moment, I started to cry. I took that person into my office, and I confessed before Him and God my sin. I confessed then to my wife, who so wonderfully and lovingly forgave me. I even told my church family, who were wholeheartedly forgiving and willing to assist in any way.

I went on the internet attempting to find a faith-based addiction program. I found the Reformers Unanimous website, and I read every detail that was available. I ordered the home study program, and I have diligently worked my way through this curriculum. It has made an amazing difference in my life. It has helped enhance my relationship with Jesus Christ. It has propelled my walk with God. I can tell you now that it has been several years since this short six-month event took place in my life, but the freedom I now experience in my personal life and ministry is intense. I've learned to give my stress and anxiety over to my Savior. I thank Him for taking that anxiety and stress upon Himself and giving me a rest deep in my soul.

Judy and Mark could not take the internal pain any longer. They saw no way to escape the pain or sense of hopelessness except through continued starvation. Like Judy and Mark, many people of all ages and walks of life battle with the seemingly invincible problem of a prescription medication addiction on a daily basis.

Does the scenario of Judy and Mark describe you or someone you love? Are you searching for answers? There are millions of people just like you or someone you know who are desperately seeking for their way out. Like Judy and Mark, many have found that way out. They were introduced to "the Way," the Lord Jesus Christ, and have joined thousands of addicts who have found freedom through this program called **Reformers Unanimous (RU)**. RU directs people to the Truth Who makes free. I speak of the Truth named the Lord Jesus Christ. Many have come to an RU meeting, facing a combination of destructive circumstances. Many have sought help on their own, like Judy and Mark, without any long-term success. Yet, these same people are transformed as they engage in the RU curriculum and participate in its extremely supportive weekly programs.

Thousands of these individuals are now productive members of society. Collectively, they are a living testimony that there is hope for you or for those whom you love.

Yes, a prescription medication addiction *(i.e., pain killers and sedative hypnotics)* CAN be eliminated from your life. There is hope! There is freedom! And, that is the gospel TRUTH!

Rx
THE TOPIC

Each prescription medication abuser knows exactly how prescription medications (such as Vicoden and Xanax) make them feel. They also recognize that the feeling it generates each time is fairly consistent. However, very few addicts actually know why it makes them feel this way, much less how it happens.

As a former cocaine addict myself, I was amazed to learn how effective drugs are at masking the real root problem in our lives. Prescription pain killers and sedatives actually manipulate neurotransmitters in the brain that create a false sense of enjoyment and calmness. This sense of enjoyment and calmness is, of course, only temporary. As well, it is not reality. However, we have a very great Creator who made our body to secrete these neurotransmitters, and He has ways of doing so without the pain and misery of prescription medication abuse.

NEUROTRANSMITTERS AND THEIR ROLES IN THE BODY:

- Acetylcholine: stimulates muscles, aids in sleep cycle
- Norepinephrine: similar to adrenaline, increases heart rate; helps form memories
- GABA (gamma-aminobutyric acid): prevents anxiety
- Glutamate: aids in memory formation
- Serotonin: regulates mood and emotion
- Endorphin: necessary for pleasure and pain reduction
- Dopamine: motivation; pleasure

In this chapter, Dr. George Crabb, a board certified Internal Medicine physician and member of the American Society of Addiction Medicine, will explain to us the phenomenon and feeling of these mood and mind-altering drugs of choice for so many.

Pain and stress are a necessary part of human life. They are warning signals indicating something is not right. Pain can be looked at as emotional pain as well as physical pain. Pain and stress are totally private. No one else can truly understand the pain or stress you feel. Pain and stress are an alarm that something is wrong and something needs to be done. In Norman

Couzen's book entitled, *Anatomy Of An Illness*, he writes "Americans are the most pain-conscious (stress conscious) people on the face of the earth." Americans have come to believe that they deserve to have total relief from their pain and stress. Because of this cultural belief, the non-medical use of prescription medications (including pain killers and sedative hypnotics) has increased dramatically over the past several years. Individuals, like Judy, take the medication for the feeling, "the high," that results from it. Although overall drug use among teenagers is down, the non-medical use of prescription medications has increased. This trend has been one of the most significant developments in substance-abuse trends in recent years. One in five teenagers has abused Vicoden, and one in ten has abused OxyContin. Both are abused for non-medical purposes.

Another reason so many are turning to prescription medications, including pain killers and sedative hypnotics, is that they feel they are safer than street drugs. This gives the user, like Judy, a false sense of security. There are a significant proportion of individuals abusing prescription medications. They believe they cannot become addicted to them like most street drugs. Individuals that use pain killers to initially treat physical pain, at times, find themselves starting to take the drug to satisfy emotional and psychological needs. The person proceeds down the road of addiction to that drug, and they have a compulsive need to use the medication for non-medical purposes. The drug is being taken because of its mood-altering effects and not to relieve the pain.

As Judy continued down her path of addiction to prescription pain killers, her behavior became erratic, as she would steal drugs from her patients as well as from family and friends. She also began to lie, obsessively count her stash of pills, and as mentioned in her testimony, she began to physician shop. She started to tell her physician that she lost her medication, it fell into the toilet, or even the ever-famous excuse, "My dog ate it!" She did it all with the goal of getting more of the drug that she most desperately needed.

Opioids are still considered one of the most highly-effective and well-tolerated of the analgesics. Analgesic is a medication that eases pain but does not cause unconsciousness. Opioids are also called "prescription narcotics." They are the most commonly-prescribed pain killers today. The opioids are derived from opium, or they can be synthesized in the laboratory with opiate-like effects. Among the most common opiates are morphine, codeine, and hydrocodone. We, in the medical field, prescribe these medications to treat moderate to severe pain and to control the pain of post-surgical patients. Codeine and hydrocodone can also be used to treat severe coughs. Morphine can be processed to produce the more rapid-acting opiate, heroin, which is sought after by millions. Methadone is yet another opiate, which is abused by many.

To understand the effects of opiates on a person's body, such as Judy, we must understand how they interact with the individual's system. Opiates attach themselves to an opiate receptor called the "mu" receptor, which is located in the brain. When an opiate attaches to the "mu" receptor, it blocks the brain's perception of pain. Because the drug affects the region of the brain with pleasure sensation, euphoria can also result. This is the feeling that Judy and so many like her began to crave. I would like to say, when these prescription opiates are taken as directed and monitored by a medical doctor, they are a safe way to manage pain in the **short term**. One of the more potent opiates is morphine. Morphine comes from the word "Morpheus," the Greek god of dreams. Heroin is actually derived from morphine. Heroin is derived from the German word "heroisch," which means "heroic." Morphine is as highly addictive as heroin. Codeine (methyl morphine) is the most widely-used, natural-occurring opiate in the world today. Codeine is commonly found in Tylenol #3 and many cough suppressants. Oxycodone is one of the strongest medications that can be taken orally for pain. It is in such mediations as Percocet and Percodan. A sustained-release form of this medicine is called OxyContin. Among the young people of our day, a new fad is to crush OxyContin and sniff the contents, achieving a high. Hydrocodone is another form of an opiate found in the derivatives of Vicoden. This is what Judy became addicted to. Like all other opiates, it attaches to the "mu" receptors in the brain and causes an intense euphoria for the user.

I had a patient in the hospital that was addicted to OxyContin. He told me that he could be happy sitting in a trash can in the dark somewhere. He went on to tell me that when he had pills, he felt like a king. He went on to explain to me that when he woke up, he snorted 30 or 40 milligrams of OxyContin to feel normal. He said, "You know, to feel normal, not sick!" The major risk associated with opioid abuse is tolerance.

Coming off of prescription pain killers should not be done on your own. Since opioids can cause sleepiness, calmness, and constipation, those addicted to opioids may experience a "revving up" of the opposite conditions. They may experience insomnia, anxiety, and diarrhea. However, the withdrawal symptoms do not stop there. Judy experienced the following:

- Restlessness
- Sweating and Chills
- Muscle and Joint Pain
- Teary Eyes
- Nasal Drainage
- Backaches
- Irritability
- Abdominal Cramps
- Nausea and Vomiting
- Increased Blood Pressure, Respiratory Rate, and Heart Rate

Judy testified to me that breaking the bonds of prescription drug addiction was the worst pain she ever felt. When she decided to break free from her addiction to Vicoden, she realized that her body must go through the process of withdrawal to rid itself of the toxic substances of the drug. She understood that how long her withdrawal symptoms would last would be dependent on what kind and how much opioids she had taken.

Not only are many people finding relief from their emotional pain by taking prescription narcotics, there is also a large group finding similar relief by partaking in a class of prescription medications called sedative hypnotics. This class of medication includes barbiturates along with the benzodiazepines. They act as depressants on the central nervous system, slowing down some of its actions. The primary medical purpose of these medications is in the treatment of certain anxiety disorders and sleep disturbances.

Stress and anxiety crosses cultural barriers and time. Each era has had its stressors: survival, war, poverty, and high-tech. Individuals throughout history have sought unhealthy methods of dealing with stress and its fallout. Some have turned to alcohol, others have turned to sedative hypnotics, and some have turned to both. But, they come with a host of problems themselves. Sedative hypnotics include all prescription sleeping medications and prescription anti-anxiety drugs. Both sedatives and hypnotics are depressants that work on the body's central nervous system slowing normal brain activity. Like most other depressants, they work on the neurotransmitter *gamma-aminobutyric acid* (GABA). GABA is an inhibitory neurotransmitter that slows action in the central nervous system. Both barbiturates and benzodiazepines increase GABA's ability in the central nervous system. In general, sedative hypnotics impair the sending and receiving of neurological impulses. They can lower blood pressure and even slow the heart rate. These medications can have a beneficial aspect in the treatment of some patients, but great care has to be given so they are not abused. As with all medications, no matter how beneficial they might be, they have side effects. Many of the side effects associated with sedative hypnotics mimic alcohol, which is another central nervous system depressant.

Some of the potential side effects of sedative hypnotics that Mark encountered were drowsiness along with impaired judgment as well as a condition called *anterograde amnesia* (forgetting events that transpired while on the medicine). Side effects can be as severe as stupor, coma, and cardiac arrest resulting in death. Mark also experienced a phenomenon while taking the sedative Xanax, which made him experience an altered perception of time and space, thus reducing sensitivity to pain. One of the more dangerous addictions that is out there is individuals taking high dosages of barbiturates mixed with alcohol. This enhances the central nervous system's depressive-effect, which, in turn, causes respiratory arrest and death. Long-term effects of the use of sedative hypnotics are as follows:

- Impaired Memory
- Impaired Judgment
- Hostility
- Depression
- Mood Swings

Another phenomenon that Mark experienced during his addiction to Xanax is called *drug automatism*. In drug automatism, someone, like Mark, who is under the influence of a sedative hypnotic (like Xanax) and who may be found in a confused state, is unaware that they have taken a dose of medication so they take another dose. This leads to a fatal overdose! Withdrawal from sedative hypnotics is quite intense. Mark describes a very horrific scene. He experienced the following withdrawal symptoms:

- Severe Anxiety
- Insomnia
- Nausea and Vomiting
- Tremors
- Intense Dizziness

- Depression
- Rapid Mood Swings

More serious side effects from sedative hypnotic withdrawal can be:

- Seizure Activity
- Visual and Auditory Hallucinations
- Tremors
- Delirium
- Paranoia
- Death

There is obviously no such thing as a "symptom free" withdrawal from sedative hypnotics. As with all other abused drugs, the withdrawal is characterized as the individual's worst nightmare. This is exactly what Mark testifies to.

The use of prescription pain killers and sedative hypnotics in a non-medical fashion is an alarming trend in drug use today, especially with our teenagers and also within our churches. A recent survey of teenagers indicated that they used prescription medications as their drug of choice because it was easily obtainable. They can find them in medicine cabinets in many homes because parents are using them. A study conducted by the National Institute on Drug Abuse (NIDA) in 2004 found that teens would gather up prescription medications, get with other teens at "pharming parties," and trade for other prescription drugs. At some parties, teens bring whatever prescription medications they find in their parent's or grandparent's medicine cabinets. They throw all the medication into a bowl, pass it around, and then take whatever they want. This is called the "salad bowl." Another reason that adults, teenagers, and church members are becoming addicted to prescription medications is that they consider them to be safer than street drugs. In a recent survey, fifty percent of those questioned did not see a major risk in taking prescription medications. They reason that these medications were prescribed by a physician (even though it was not meant for them) and are permitted by the law. However, these individuals are using them and abusing them for non-medical purposes.

Individuals who use illegal drugs often use sedative hypnotics, especially barbiturates. Individuals who use heroin combine it with barbiturates to get a more intense high. However, since both barbiturates and heroin depress respiration, this can be an extremely dangerous and deadly practice. Methamphetamine users also combine their drug of choice with barbiturates. When someone uses methamphetamine over a course of several days, they experience severe hyperactivity. To counteract this hyperactivity, some methamphetamine users will take sedative hypnotics. According to the Drug Enforcement Agency (DEA), an estimated fifty percent of people who undergo treatment for narcotic or cocaine addiction report abusing benzodiazepines or barbiturates.

All that Judy, Mark, and the other millions of individuals in our society today are looking for is help to heal the hurt that lives down deep within them.

Friend, regardless of where you may be in your struggle with a prescription medication addiction, the good news is that there is life after your addiction. Judy and Mark found this life. For this to be accomplished in your life, there must be a change in your behavior. I want you to know that the only effective way of changing your behavior is changing the beliefs to which you hold. This will be the subject of the remainder of this book.

STEROIDS

STEROIDS
The Testimony

Joshua's Testimony

As a young man, I as already addicted to prescription medications, but I learned of something "new," steroids. It was a hard thing to find, but with the right connection, I was well on my way. It was actually through one of my brother's friends that I got "turned on" to steroids. I recall seeing this guy, how muscular he was, and thinking to myself, "Is that humanly possible?" My first meeting with him was pretty to the point. It all boiled down to, CAN YOU GET ME SOME STEROIDS? To my surprise, it was very easy.

I was married at the time and remember taking pills at first (they were called DBOL). I took three pills a day and noticed within a week my attitude changed, my moods changed, I was much more angry, and I was more agitated and edgy. I joined a gym and began working out. I did it because I was a small-framed guy, five foot seven and about 167 pounds. Within a month, I gained 15 pounds. By the time the pills ran out, I felt that I needed more. Not only did I need more, but I wanted something better. That is when I was introduced to injectable steroids. I really did not like needles, but I got over that fear really quick. My justification of doing steroids is that our body makes its own steroids, so I am just putting more into my body so it will grow faster. Along with my steroid addiction came an eating addiction. I was eating eight times a day. The crazy part is that you usually take a steroid cycle and quit (on a month and off a month), but I never quit. My marriage started to deteriorate. I went from a very good, loving husband to going to work and then directly to the gym. I lived for the gym. What about my wife? I mean I loved my wife, but the addiction to steroids was so strong that it came down to the gym. I would rather lift weights than be with my wife. I do remember, after using steroids once, I woke up with my lower leg swollen so big it looked like a football. The physician said that I could have possibly lost it. Did that stop me? Absolutely not! I took the medication the physician gave me to take care of my leg and went right back to using steroids.

Everything else, addiction wise, grew strong in my life. Prescription pills everyday and then other drugs. I eventually got caught. I was pulled over by the police, and they went through my duffle bag and found a two years' supply of steroids. That was enough to get me arrested for being a seller. It turned out that this was a blessing from God. God was opening the door for me to have a chance to escape this bondage and find glorious freedom in His Son, Jesus Christ. While I was in jail, my wife wrote me a letter. She said that she hired a divorce attorney and wanted out. Do you blame her? It was the worst feeling I had ever went through. All during the prison time of my life (about six years), never was I completely at rock bottom. One month in jail and divorce papers in my hands finally landed me at rock bottom. The grief I felt inside tore me apart. God allowed me to get out of jail on probation, and then I went and slapped Him in the face by using steroids again.

Thank God, though, I found Reformers Unanimous through my home church. The relief I felt knowing God could and did forgive me brought me so much freedom. I finally found freedom from my addiction. My life is changing daily. God is filling my heart and spirit daily. I no longer have pride deep in my life. I cry when I want because my God allows me to feel feelings. God is so good to me.

I now have a job working with my Reformers Unanimous director. I have family support. Not only that, the emptiness I had been feeling for the last year and a half has been filled by God with joy and happiness. God blessed me enough to not only die for me, but He put Christian people into my life through Reformers Unanimous.

Joshua could not take the internal pain any longer. He saw no way to escape the pain or sense of hopelessness except through continued use of steroids. Like Joshua, many people of all ages and walks of life battle with the seemingly invincible problem of steroid addiction on a daily basis.
Does the scenario of Joshua describe you or someone you love? Are you searching for answers? There are millions of people just like you or someone you know who are desperately seeking for their way out. Like Joshua, many have found that way out. They were introduced to "the Way," the Lord Jesus Christ, and have joined thousands of addicts who have found freedom through this program called **Reformers Unanimous (RU)**. RU directs people to the Truth Who makes free. I speak of the Truth named the Lord Jesus Christ. Many have come to an RU meeting, facing a combination of destructive circumstances. Many have sought help on their own, like Joshua, without any long-term success. Yet, these same people

are transformed as they engage in the RU curriculum and participate in its extremely supportive weekly programs.

Thousands of these individuals are now productive members of society. Collectively, they are a living testimony that there is hope for you or for those whom you love.

Yes, steroids CAN be eliminated from your life. There is hope! There is freedom! And, that is the gospel TRUTH!

STEROIDS
THE TOPIC

Each steroid user knows exactly how steroids make them feel. They also recognize that the feeling it generates each time is fairly consistent. However, very few abusers actually know why it makes them feel this way, much less how it happens.

As with all other addictive drugs, it is amazing to learn how effective they are at masking the real root problem in a person's life. Steroids actually manipulate neurotransmitters in the brain that create a false sense of well being. This sense of pleasure and calmness is, of course, only temporary. As well, it is not reality. However, we have a very great Creator who made our body to secrete these neurotransmitters, and He has ways of doing so without the pain and misery of steroid abuse.

NEUROTRANSMITTERS AND THEIR ROLES IN THE BODY:

- Acetylcholine: stimulates muscles, aids in sleep cycle
- Norepinephrine: similar to adrenaline, increases heart rate; helps form memories
- GABA (gamma-aminobutyric acid): prevents anxiety
- Glutamate: aids in memory formation
- Serotonin: regulates mood and emotion
- Endorphin: necessary for pleasure and pain reduction
- Dopamine: motivation; pleasure

In this chapter, Dr. George Crabb, a board certified Internal Medicine physician and member of the American Society of Addiction Medicine, will explain to us the phenomenon and feeling of this mood and mind-altering drug of choice for so many.

Joshua was not happy with the way he looked. At first glance, one might assume that if we are reading about someone who is unhappy about their appearance, it must be a female. This is not always the case. Guys, like Joshua, choose an unhealthy way to improve their appearance – STEROIDS!

Steroids are naturally-occurring hormones in the body. Although all steroids are lipids composed of a carbon skeleton with four fused rings attached, steroids differ in what functions are attached to the rings. In the human body, steroids act as hormones. When steroids attach to steroid-receptor proteins, cells adapt to fight stress, promote growth, and bring on puberty. Those are the naturally-occurring steroids and not the type that Joshua used to enhance his appearance.

Now, the steroids that Joshua used are the synthetic ones called anabolic androgenic steroids. Anabolic refers to their muscle-building properties, and androgenic referring to their ability to increase masculine characteristics. In the case of anabolic androgenic steroids, often just called anabolic steroids, the word, steroid, indicates the class of drugs. The anabolic steroids that Joshua was taking were synthetic derivatives of testosterone, the sex hormone. Testosterone is the most important androgen. Testosterone can affect not only certain male characteristics of the body, but they can also affect how aggressive someone is. Although steroids have often been in the news for the past several years, they are not a new discovery. And, neither is the desire to perform and look better. Unless we forget, females also abuse steroids. They use them to lose weight and tone up.

Originally, steroid abuse was most often found on college campuses and in Olympic and professional sports. Today, most steroid abuse continues to occur among athletes, professional and amateur. According to the American Academy of Pediatrics, steroid abuse is most likely to occur within these groups. Athletes involved in sports that rely on strength and size are the football, wrestling, or baseball athletes, and endurance athletes are those that are involved in track and field, swimming, weight training, or body building.

According to the website, www.coolnurse.com, teens feel pressured to use steroids because of the "nots" in their lives. For them, they have reasons to abuse steroids, such as:

- Not making the sports team
- Not meeting peer pressures and demands
- Not getting the "girls"
- Not able to compete with others who are using steroids
- Not looking as good as you could

The pressure that these individuals feel can transcend the present. All that matters is how they feel and look at the moment and not about the long-term consequences of steroid use.

And, again, athletes are not the only ones taking steroids. Others take steroids to increase their muscle mass and decrease their amount of body fat. Although this may include many athletes, it just as easily includes individuals who simply want to look better, i.e., a guy who wants more muscles so he will be more attractive, and a girl who wants a more toned look. Individuals who abuse steroids, like Joshua, for these reasons, have a distorted body image. The reality of how they look is opposite of what is perceived. Others who use steroids to increase muscle mass have experienced some kind of abuse – usually either physically or sexual and when they were often very young.

Female weight lifters who used steroids or other body-enhancing substances were twice as likely to have been raped than their non-steroid using peer. Most females who abuse steroids do so to reduce body fat and increase muscles. Many of them have a concurrent eating disorder.

Today, there are ten major classes of anabolic steroids, based on how they are taken into the body and the carrier-solvent that introduces the steroid into the body. The classes are:

1. Oral
2. Injectable Oil Based
3. Injectable Water Based
4. Transdermal Patch or Gel
5. Aerosol Propellant-Based Preparation
6. Sub-lingual
7. Homemade Transdermal Preparation
8. Androgen/Estrogen Combination
9. Counterfeit Anabolic
10. Over-The-Counter

Despite their known dangers and the fact that they are controlled substances, obtaining the above steroids can be relatively easy. The internet is an easy source to go to when wanting to obtain steroids.

Most individuals who abuse steroids have a very distinctive pattern to their usage. Many use a **"cycling"** pattern, which means they use steroids over a specific period, stopping for a while, and then starting the process over again. And, then, there are individuals, like Joshua, that continued to take steroids on a daily basis with no cessation at all. **"Stacking"** is another popular way of taking steroids. This pattern involves taking several different types of steroids, usually mixing ingestible and injectable types of the drugs. In some cases, individuals use steroids developed for use in veterinary medicine. Individuals who "stack" their steroids believe that the mixing of the steroids increase their ultimate effect. They think they will get better results than if they used the individual steroids alone. When abusers **"pyramid,"** they slowly increase how much or how often (or both) they take steroids. Many also include "stacking" in their pyramid routine. They often operate on a cycle of six to twelve weeks. At first, the dosage is low. Gradually, dosage and frequency increase until they reach a peek during the mid-point of the cycle. Abusers, then, start tapering off the dosage until they are no longer taking steroids. When this point is reached, individuals usually spend some time completely off steroids before resuming another "pyramid" cycle.

Joshua said in his testimony that he believed he was never big enough, and that is why he continued to escalate his steroid use. He also went on to tell me in a private conversation, "I was almost like a heroin addict!" He said it got to the point where he needed the injection to work out and feel good about himself.

Anger is just one of the possible side effects of taking steroids. Some of the side effects are classified relatively minor, such as:

- Acne
- Oily Hair
- Purple or Red Spots on the Body
- Legs and Feet Swelling
- Bad Breath

Joshua's appetite increased, and because of the steroid use, his bone marrow became stimulated into producing more red blood cells. This increases the risk of stroke and heart attack. Other potential side effects are far more serious and include the possibility of death. Steroids affect all areas of the human body. Steroids affect the endocrine system. In men, this can demonstrate as male-pattern baldness and gynecomastia, which is the increase of an individual's breasts. In women, they will develop male characteristics. Women's skin will become rougher, and for some women, they will develop baldness and hair on their body will increase. They will even experience a deeper voice. The steroids can also affect the cardiovascular system, increasing the risk of heart attacks and strokes. Steroid use can result in elevated blood pressure, as Joshua is aware of. Steroid use also increases the possibility of blood clots forming in the blood vessels. The effects of steroid abuse on the liver can be deadly. Liver tumors and a rare condition called *peliosis hepatis* have been found in people with a history of steroid abuse. This is a condition where cysts filled with blood form in the liver. Should liver tumors or the cysts of *peliosis hepatis* rupture, internal bleeding can occur and lead to death.

Steroids can also affect behavior and increase aggression, also a condition known as *roid rage*. According to the National Institute of Drug Abuse, 2006, some individuals who abused steroids reported that they committed physical violence: robbery, theft, vandalism, or burglary. They admitted that they were more apt to commit these crimes while on steroids. Mania, delusions, and depression have also been reported in individuals who abuse steroids.

Another side effect of abusing steroids, as was with Joshua, is co-addiction to other drugs. In many cases, the additional drug is taken to alleviate some of the potential, adverse effects of the steroids. A NIDA, 2006, study of 227 men undergoing inpatient treatment for heroin or other opioid abuse, found that 9.3 percent of them had started their illicit drug use by abusing anabolic steroids. Of those, 86 percent used the opioids to treat the insomnia and rage they had as a side effect of taking steroids.

Some individuals, like Joshua, no matter how bad the side effects are or how dire the outlook caused by their steroid abuse, they just won't or can't stop. When Joshua finally broke free from his addition to steroids, he went into a deep depression while withdrawing. He told me, "It was like coming down off a high, and I started getting really depressed." Other symptoms that Joshua observed during his withdrawal syndrome included:

- **Drastic Mood Swings**
- **Fatigue**
- **Restlessness**
- **Loss of Appetite**
- **Insomnia**
- **Craving for the Steroid**

But, again, the most serious symptom is depression. In some cases that I have dealt with in my clinic, the individuals had suicidal thoughts. I have had some patients that actually attempted suicide, and I have known of some that were successful in their suicide attempts.

Because of the long, lingering affect of steroids on the body, some symptoms of the depression can linger for more than a year after the person stops taking the steroids.

REMEMBER: Overcoming steroid addiction is no different than with every other form of addiction.

All that Joshua and the other millions of individuals in our society today are looking for is help to heal the hurt that lives down deep within them.

Friend, regardless of where you may be in your struggle with steroid addiction, the good news is that there is life after steroids. Joshua found this life. For this to be accomplished in your life, there must be a change in your behavior. I want you to know that the only effective way of changing your behavior is changing the beliefs to which you hold. This will be the subject of the remainder of this book.

TOBACCO

Ken's Testimony

Hi, my name is Ken. I am sixty-five years old. I believe I had as about a normal childhood as anyone could. I had a loving father and mother who were Christians. They guided me and my brother and sister into things of God. We were faithful to church services on Sunday and Wednesday night. Anytime there were special events going on at the church, our family was present. My parents supported and encouraged me and were always there for me no matter what. I accepted Jesus Christ as my Savior as a teenager. I was baptized, and I read my Bible and prayed almost every day. I enjoyed reading my Bible. I enjoyed the facts about all the special events in the Old Testament as well as the events surrounding the life of Jesus and the apostles. My family and my friends always commented to me on the vast knowledge base that I had regarding the Word of God. Even though I knew much about the Bible, I looked at it as more of an academic issue than a relationship issue with my Savior, Jesus Christ.

I was drafted into the army after high school. During my time in the military, I felt a lot of stress and frustration. I did not have my family to fall back on, and I did not have a good local church to attend and receive support from. Most of my buddies in the army smoked cigarettes. For a while, as they offered a cigarette to me, I would refuse. However, after a while, I did try one. As I tried that first cigarette, it made me feel very good. It made my stress level less, and it seemed that my frustrations vanished. Over the next two years in the army, my cigarette smoking escalated to almost two packs per day. I almost viewed the ritual of smoking as a friend, a friend that I could turn to almost anytime that would make me feel good, help me deal with my stress and frustration, and it was a friend that would not criticize, judge, or talk back. All along, however, I knew that my cigarette use was not glorifying to God let alone healthy. As I returned to civilian life and to my family, friends, and local church, I initially kept my cigarette use a secret. As time went on, the veil of secrecy was slowly torn away, and it was common knowledge that I was a smoker. There were several positions that my pastor asked me to fill in our church. But, I knew I could not properly serve in those areas because of my cigarette habit. Once I was asked to become a Deacon of our church, but I had to refuse the position. I cannot tell you how devastating that was to me. I knew what I was doing was wrong. It was not glorifying God, and it was destroying my body and hindering my testimony. I attempted to quit on several occasions with all ending in failure. On one occasion, I was able to go without cigarettes for twenty days, and I thought I had beaten the problem. Then, though, a stressful situation arose in our family, and I turned to cigarettes for relief. After approximately forty years of nicotine addiction, I was basically a broken man. I knew God did not want me to continue with this habit, but I did not know how to stop.

One Sunday evening, while sitting in the pew at church, awaiting my pastor's message, he made an announcement that our church was going to start an addiction program on Friday nights. With great interest, I listened as he explained the program. I remember going home that evening after the Sunday night service, lying across my bed, crying and thanking God that He had led our pastor to start this program. I went to see my physician, who gave me some medical advice and help regarding the stoppage of my cigarette addiction and wholeheartedly dove in to the Reformers Unanimous Program. I began to journal daily in the Reformers Unanimous Daily Journal. As I went through the "Strongholds" course, I realized that, although the academic knowledge of the Word of God is vital, the most vital part is a relationship with Jesus Christ. As I looked back on this addiction to nicotine that tormented me for forty years, I finally realized that what I needed and desired was a relationship with Jesus Christ and not a substitute drug.

I can now tell you that for the past three years I have not had one cigarette. I walk in the freedom that Jesus purchased for me through His death, burial, and resurrection. When times of stress and frustration enter my life, I now know that instead of turning to nicotine I turn to my Savior, my Friend, who will meet every need. I thank God on a daily basis for the deliverance He has given to me and will certainly give to you if you will walk with Him.

Ken could not take the internal pain any longer. He saw no way to escape the pain or sense of hopelessness except through continued use of tobacco. Like Ken, many people of all ages and walks of life battle with the seemingly invincible problem of nicotine addiction on a daily basis.

Does the scenario of Ken describe you or someone you love? Are you searching for answers? There are millions of people just like you or someone you know who are desperately seeking for their way out. Like Ken, many have found that way out. They were introduced to "the Way," the Lord Jesus Christ, and have joined thousands of addicts who have found freedom through this program called **Reformers Unanimous (RU)**. RU directs people to the Truth Who makes free. I speak of the Truth named the Lord Jesus Christ. Many have come to an RU meeting, facing a combination of destructive circumstances. Many have sought help on their own, like Ken, without any long-term success. Yet, these same people are transformed as they engage in the RU curriculum and participate in its extremely supportive weekly programs.

Thousands of these individuals are now productive members of society. Collectively, they are a living testimony that there is hope for you or for those whom you love.

Yes, tobacco CAN be eliminated from your life. There is hope! There is freedom! And, that is the gospel TRUTH!

TOBACCO
THE TOPIC

Each tobacco user knows exactly how nicotine makes them feel. They also recognize that the feeling it generates each time is fairly consistent. However, very few smokers actually know why it makes them feel this way, much less how it happens.

As with all other addictive drugs, it is amazing to learn how effective they are at masking the real root problem in a person's life. Nicotine actually acts on a specific type of neurotransmitter called acetylcholine that creates a false sense of enjoyment. This sense of pleasure is, of course, only temporary. As well, it is not reality. However, we have a very great Creator who made our body to secrete these neurotransmitters, and He has ways of doing so without the pain and misery of tobacco abuse.

NEUROTRANSMITTERS AND THEIR ROLES IN THE BODY:

- Acetylcholine: stimulates muscles, aids in sleep cycle
- Norepinephrine: similar to adrenaline, increases heart rate; helps form memories
- GABA (gamma-aminobutyric acid): prevents anxiety
- Glutamate: aids in memory formation
- Serotonin: regulates mood and emotion
- Endorphin: necessary for pleasure and pain reduction
- Dopamine: motivation; pleasure

In this chapter, Dr. George Crabb, a board certified Internal Medicine physician and member of the American Society of Addiction Medicine, will explain to us the phenomenon and feeling of this mood and mind-altering drug of choice for so many.

Ken, who we read about earlier, experienced the effect of a chemical found in the tobacco plant (*Nicotiana tabacum*), which is native to North and South America. This specific type of tobacco plant is widely cultivated for cigarette use because its leaves produce mild smoke. Tobacco, with its drug, nicotine, is probably the most widely abused chemical substance in the world. It is one of the most difficult addictions to conquer. Young people are especially at risk. For many teenagers believe they can smoke for a few years and quit. This is rarely the case. Cigarettes are designed to addict. They are chemically engineered to deliver nicotine to your brain. Ken, as most other individuals that smoke cigarettes, was unaware of the many dangerous chemicals they are inhaling. As Ken inhaled the cigarette smoke, he was also inhaling acetone (found in paint stripper) as well as carbon monoxide (found in car exhaust fumes), along with many other toxic gases, including hydrogen cyanide and formaldehyde. In the cigarette smoke is also nicotine, the naturally-occurring chemical (drug) in tobacco that makes smoking addictive. The many unnatural chemicals added to tobacco make the cigarette even more deadly. These added chemicals are given the general name "tar" and include everything in a cigarette but nicotine and water. The cigarette is manufactured with a deadly delivery system, designed to efficiently send high doses of nicotine to the brain. As you inhale the cigarette smoke, the tar infiltrates your lungs, and the nicotine rides the "tar" into the blood stream. As Ken inhaled the cigarette smoke, there were over four thousand compounds present in that smoke to make that "rush" of nicotine faster and more enjoyable. Out of the over four thousand compounds present in cigarette smoke, at least sixty of them are known to be carcinogens (cancer-forming chemicals).

I have had many patients tell me, "Cigarettes are the only dangerous source of tobacco." These individuals are under a false impression. They believe that other tobacco products are less dangerous than cigarettes. This certainly is a lie. In fact, cigars can deliver as much tar and nicotine as a pack or more of cigarettes, thus, exposing the individual and those around them. Second-hand smoke has very high levels of disease-causing poison. We, therefore, conclude that cigar smoke is every bit as poisonous and dangerous as cigarette smoke.

Another source of tobacco that I am confronted with in my practice is smokeless tobacco. Smokeless tobacco is another dangerous substance. Snuff, chewing tobacco, and gutka (a mix of lime paste, areca nut, spices, and tobacco sealed inside plastic or foil) are three popular forms of smokeless tobacco. The dangers associated with smokeless tobacco are nicotine addiction just like the smoked tobacco, but also, a significantly increased risk of oral cancers.

Tobacco is quite insidious with its consequences. Unlike cocaine, heroin, or other dangerous drugs, tobacco's nicotine and poison can go undetected for many years. Tobacco can gradually create addiction to nicotine and gradually kill. Tobacco is legal and accessible, but it is one of the leading causes of death throughout the world, causing almost half a million deaths in the United States annually.

As Ken continued his forty year addiction with nicotine, he was not only exposing himself to the dangers of tobacco but also his loved ones and friends who he smoked around. As Ken would light a cigarette, the fumes from the lit cigarette that would go into the air along with the exhaled smoke from Ken's lungs is called second-hand smoke. Second-hand smoke was once considered not hazardous, but we now know better. We now understand that smoking is a practice that also affects those around you. When you smoke, you don't just inhale all the toxins and nicotine that we discussed earlier, but you exhale them into the air around you. Not only do you exhale these poisons, but the smoke released from a lit cigarette (tobacco product) contains toxins as well. This second-hand smoke is poisonous and it kills. When Ken's wife inhaled smoke from his cigarette, she inhaled the same poisons Ken was inhaling when he smoked, which put her at risk for the very same diseases the actual smoker can contract. It is estimated that exposure to second-hand smoke causes an estimated three thousand lung cancer deaths each year among non-smoking American adults.

Tobacco has had an enormous impact on our culture. I know that tobacco has had an enormous impact on Ken's life by listening to his testimony. The whole process started in Ken's life with a substance called nicotine. There are no if's, and's, or maybe's about it...NICOTINE IS ADDICTIVE! A smoker's body, like Ken's, does not adjust to nicotine, it develops a craving for it. Ken, along with all other smokers, gain an increasing tolerance for nicotine, requiring more cigarettes and smoke to satisfy their cravings. Nicotine became a part of Ken's body's chemistry and eventually, as is the case with heroin or cocaine addicts, his body does not feel normal anymore without nicotine in his system.

It does not stop there! Cigarettes' additive qualities may also result from a by product of tobacco smoke called acetaldehyde. It has been demonstrated scientifically that when nicotine is combined with acetaldehyde, it is three times as addictive. This is a deadly combination found in every cigarette. Nicotine, itself, is a deadly chemical. In fact, fifty milligrams of pure nicotine on an individual's tongue can kill instantly. Another interesting fact that Ken was unaware of is that nicotine is so deadly that farmers use it as an insecticide to protect their crops.

The following is how cigarettes delivered nicotine to Ken's body:

Nicotine and cigarette smoke reaches the lung's alveoli (air sacs in the lungs), where it is rapidly absorbed into the bloodstream, often in as little as seven seconds. Then, the blood carries the nicotine to the brain. The process is fast and extremely effective. In fact, smoked nicotine reaches the brain more quickly than heroin injected into the veins with a needle.

The above process which I just described is devastating. I believe that part of the devastation is that we, as a society, have minimized the addictive potential of nicotine. When, in fact, studies have showed that, milligram for milligram, nicotine is five to ten times more potent than cocaine. We must reiterate this to ourselves and our children that nicotine is an addictive drug and as powerful in many ways as cocaine and heroin and causes much more death, destruction, and disease.

Once Ken inhaled the smoke from his cigarette (for others maybe a cigar), the nicotine reached his brain in only a few seconds. Once in the brain, the nicotine affected the communication between Ken's brain cells called neurons. Nicotine acts on a specific type of neurotransmitter called acetylcholine, which delivers signals from your brain to your muscles. This neurotransmitter controls your:

- Energy Level
- Heart Rate
- Respiration (how often you take a breath)
- Flow of Information
- Learning Ability
- Memory

As nicotine entered into Ken's brain, it increased the amount of acetylcholine, which increased the amount of messages transmitted between his brains cells. This caused an almost immediate feeling of alertness, rise in energy level, and what seemed like an increased ability to pay attention or focus.

Nicotine also caused the increase of a second neurotransmitter in Ken's brain called dopamine. Dopamine works on the part of the brain responsible for motivation, happy feelings, and pleasurable sensations. Dopamine is the same neurotransmitter affected by highly-addictive drugs like heroin, cocaine, and methamphetamine. When the dopamine level increased in Ken's brain, it made him feel more peaceful. The situation he was in would be more pleasurable and calm.

In addition to manipulating the neurotransmitters acetylcholine and dopamine, nicotine also caused an increase production of endorphins in Ken's brain. Endorphins are our bodies' natural pain-killing proteins. These natural analgesics (pain killers) can cause feelings of euphoria, like a "runner's high." It can also reduce the awareness of pain. Ken would tell you that what kept bringing him back to cigarettes was the feeling of more pleasure and less pain. This was a direct result of nicotine's effect on endorphins.

The downside of nicotine is that the effect on the brain does not last. Ken's brain would cry out for more nicotine as soon as thirty minutes of finishing a cigarette. The good feelings supplied to Ken by nicotine are short lived. This required Ken to use tobacco products more and more to get the same high. Another downside to nicotine is that some of the neurotransmitters responsible for nicotine's energetic feelings or short term highs are the same neurotransmitters involved in anxiety and depression. Many smokers like Ken become more prone to anxiety, panic attacks, and agoraphobia (fear of public places).

And, in fact, when we look at the effects of nicotine on the brain in regards to teenagers, smoking was the single strongest predictor of a teenager developing depressive symptoms.

Nicotine did not only affect Ken's brain, it worked on other areas of his body. Nicotine caused Ken's body to release a hormone called adrenaline. This made his heart beat faster, his breathing rate to increase, and his blood pressure to rise. While nicotine caused a release of adrenaline, it also blocked another hormone called insulin. Too little insulin results in higher levels of sugar in your blood, a condition called hyperglycemia. Thus, your body cuts back on its desire for food. This causes the reduced appetite that Ken experienced.

The long-term effects of tobacco use are devastating. Smoking is the number one cause of preventable illness. Cancers, caused by tobacco, can occur nearly anywhere in the body. The most common tobacco-related cancers occur in the:

- Mouth
- Throat
- Lungs

Let me share with you how this addiction harms your body:

- Increased Stroke Risk
- Heart Attacks
- Poor Circulation (peripheral vascular disease)
- Diabetes
- Spine & Hip Fractures
- Osteoporosis
- Premature Aging of Skin
- Blindness (macular degeneration)
- Cataracts
- Aortic Aneurysms
- Stomach Ulcers
- Pneumonia
- Sense of Smell Damage
- Longer Wound Healing
- Discoloration of Teeth
- Longer Surgical Recovery
- Gum Disease
- Weakened Immune System
- Reduced Sense of Taste
- Bad Breath
- Chronic Cough
- Emphysema
- Shortness of Breath
- Multiple Cancers, such as:
  - Liver - Pancreas
  - Kidney - Lung
  - Bladder - Colon
  - Esophagus - Stomach

Lung cancer is the most common cancer associated with smoking. Nearly ninety percent of all lung cancers are caused by smoking. Death from lung cancer is a long, slow suffocation that can take months or even years. Ken, today, suffers from many medical conditions that were at least in part caused or exacerbated by his tobacco abuse. Ken has had a heart attack, suffers from severe peripheral arterial disease (decreased blood flow to his legs), and his peripheral arterial disease is so severe that it limits his ability to walk any long distances without severe cramping in his legs. He also suffers from a moderate degree of emphysema, causing shortness of breath. Ken looks back on his forty years of nicotine addiction and wishes that it was never a part of his life. But, thankfully, Ken has stopped, and he would tell us that, even after forty years and the consequences he suffers from this destructive behavior, it was still worth quitting at this late stage in his life.

As Ken made the commitment to break the bondage of his nicotine addiction, he knew that the nicotine had actually changed his brain's chemical makeup. He knew he would go through nicotine withdrawal. For you see, when you take nicotine away, your body craves it, and it makes you feel like you need more nicotine or you will die or get sick. Your body will rebel with all kinds of symptoms:

- **Headaches**
- **Anxiety**
- **Depression (dysphoric moods)**
- **Fatigue**
- **Hunger (weight gain)**
- **Trouble Sleeping (insomnia)**
- **Thirst**
- **Trouble Paying Attention**
- **Agitation (restlessness)**
- **Irritability**
- **Jitters**
- **Feelings of Anger**
- **Difficulty Concentrating**
- **Feelings of Frustration**

The above symptoms can occur in just a few short hours after your last cigarette. They will be at their worst two to three days later and can last for weeks.

Ken testified to me that his withdrawal symptoms were so bad at times that he felt like he had no other choice but to smoke to ease his discomfort. Ken did not choose to smoke again, but this is why so many people try to quit and fail. It is not only a physical withdrawal from nicotine that a smoker goes through. In quitting tobacco, there is physiological and emotional changes that occur. For you see, smokers just don't depend on nicotine physically. They depend on it behaviorally and psychologically.

Smoking was the thing Ken did when he got together with his friends. And, in fact, it was a major means in Ken's life to blow off steam when he was feeling tense, whether with the family or at work. It was what Ken did when he drank his morning coffee or relaxed after dinner. That is why breaking the bondage of nicotine addiction can be difficult and, in fact, can be harder to quit in some instances than heroin or cocaine. A patient of mine that was involved in polysubstance abuse (including tobacco) stated to me, "It (tobacco) was the hardest to quit, and it was the last to leave." He went on to say, "The thoughts of tobacco use still haunt me." But, breaking the bondage to your nicotine addiction is of vital importance for you and those around you. Breaking this bondage is well worth the effort.

Within twenty minutes after Ken smoked his last cigarette, his body began a series of changes that have continued and will continue for years to come. Twenty minutes after his last cigarette, Ken's heart rate dropped. Twelve hours after his last cigarette, his carbon monoxide level in his blood dropped to normal. Two weeks to three months after his last cigarette, Ken's heart attack risk dropped and his lung functions improved. (Ken's heart attack occurred during his active addiction to nicotine.) One to nine months after Ken's last cigarette, his coughing and shortness of breath decreased. At Ken's one year anniversary, his added risk of coronary heart disease is half that of a current smoker. When Ken reaches his five year anniversary, his stroke risk will be reduced to that of a non smoker. When he reaches his ten year anniversary, his lung cancer death rate will approach about half of that of a non-smoker's death rate. Ken's risk of cancer of the mouth, throat, kidney, bladder, pancreas, and esophagus also significantly decreases. And, Lord willing, if Ken reaches his fifteenth anniversary, his risk of coronary heart disease is back to that of a non smoker's.

So, we see the significance of breaking the bondage of nicotine/tobacco addiction. It is so important from the physical side as well as the mental side, but also, and even more importantly, from the Spiritual side as Ken's testimony demonstrates. That is why I educate my patients that attend the Reformers Unanimous Program that instead of picking up a cigarette with your morning coffee, pick up your Bible and read it. Instead of lighting up a cigarette on your drive home, put in a preaching CD or a Joy Belle music CD. Instead of lighting up a cigarette after dinner, take a walk and meditate on the things of God.

Friend, regardless of where you may be in your struggle with nicotine addiction, the good news is that there is life after cigarettes. Ken found this life. For this to be accomplished in your life, there must be a change in your behavior. I want you to know that the only effective way of changing your behavior is changing the beliefs to which you hold. This will be the subject of the remainder of this book.

UPPERS

UPPERS
THE TESTIMONIES

Jacob's Testimony

I started using Ritalin when I was in college. I was taking a full load of courses as well as working a full-time job. I started to see my grades slip because I was unable to maintain my focus on my studies. I was talking to one of my friends regarding this problem, and he pulled out of his pocket a prescription bottle of Ritalin. He told me that he was diagnosed with ADHD as a teenager and that he was given Ritalin by his physician. He went on to tell me that it helped him stay focused and have more energy so that he could accomplish his school work and maintain a job as well. He offered me some, and I immediately took it. I knew that I could not continue with my full-time job and a full load of courses without some help. Initially, I found the help I needed. It helped me stay focused. I felt that my concentration was fine tuned. I found that I could rebound after a big night out. Down deep, I acknowledged to myself that it was probably not a good thing to do, but I did need it to get a "leg up" in my pursuit of a career. Even though I grew up in a Christian home, I put all that aside when I entered the college scene.

I soon began to take Ritalin not only for the increased focus and concentration, but I started to take it because of the "high" feeling that it gave me. My use of Ritalin escalated quite rapidly. I would have to take at least 40 milligrams in the morning just to get me started. When my supply of Ritalin ran out and I was unable to secure any, I would start slipping into a deep depression. The depression was so severe at times I contemplated suicide. During winter break in my junior year of college, I went home to spend a few days with my family. I had underestimated how much Ritalin I would need during that short trip, therefore, I ran out. I fell into a deep depression. Laying there in my old bedroom, I took a handful of Tylenol P.M. in an attempt to stop my pain. My parents found me, saw what I had done, and they called 911. The ambulance took me to the emergency room where the physician on call pumped my stomach and gave me certain medicines in an attempt to counteract the overdose. I was in the hospital for several weeks recovering from my suicide attempt. During that time, my loving parents and my wonderful pastor of my church visited me and offered help in any way. During those few weeks, I was able to share with them the mess I had made of my life. My parents and pastor helped during that period of time, and they directed me to a program called Reformers Unanimous. This was a Friday night addiction program that actually started at my local church during my freshman year at college. I started to attend those Friday night meetings, and I was reacquainted with my Savior, Jesus Christ. All along, I was attempting to manage and control my own life when what I really needed to be doing was placing my life under the control of my loving, heavenly Father.

I moved back home and enrolled in a local college as to stay near my parents, church, and the RU help I was receiving. This also relieved the financial burden because I was able to live at home. I became faithful to my church as well as the RU program. I put myself under the authority of my pastor and parents once again. I can tell you now that I lead an exciting, exuberant life with no need of an outside source such as Ritalin. I have found all I need in my Savior, Jesus Christ.

Justin's Testimony

I started taking Adderall after I got out of prison for manufacturing methamphetamine. I was addicted to methamphetamine for a little over three years. That is all I wanted, and it did not matter how much it cost. The fact is that I loved the feeling I got when high on speed. A friend turned me on to "addies" one day, and said, "It is just like methamphetamine only without the hard come down." So, we crushed up two, 30 milligram capsules and snorted a big line. In about 15 minutes I was going about 120 miles per hour. Well, my friend lied to me. There was a big come down for me after a four-day binge and a full prescription of 60, 30 milligram pills. I felt the big come down. After that, it was just like my methamphetamine addiction. I wanted more Adderall, and I wanted it everyday. I started taking my cousin's prescription, something that he really needed. However, my selfishness did not care about what he needed. I said, "So what if he needs it medically. I need it also!" I traded my wife's medicine for addies and then tried to hide it from her. I would go to where my sister was and beg her to give me some. I remember offering her two or three hundred dollars for 30 pills. I was like that for about one year before I switched my addiction to OxyContin. For me to be speeding was a way of life. I felt that I could not do anything unless I had Adderall. I thought it made me a better and productive person. I felt that I could not do anything or finish anything without being high. The truth of the matter was that I could not finish anything. I would start something, and I was going so fast, having too many things going on at once, that nothing truly ever got done. Whether it was pills, speed, weed, acid, or heroin, the truth was that I was too busy looking for the next high to ever complete anything.

When I was arrested this time, I knew there had to be something different. Something had to change, and I could not do it on my own. Believe me, I had tried three other times to quit. God needed to be in my life. I prayed two years ago in a prison cell for God to help me understand His will for me, and I wanted to have patience enough to sit down and read His Word. I prayed for God to get closer to me and for Him to direct my path. Well, my prayer was answered! I am now sitting here in Reformers Unanimous where I have nothing but time to concentrate on my Heavenly Father. I was foolish to think I could kick my addiction on my own. I know now that I can do nothing without God. I want to thank my Heavenly Father that He brought a program like Reformers Unanimous in my life so that I may have a chance at real life.

Jacob and Justin could not take the internal pain any longer. They saw no way to escape the pain or sense of hopelessness except through continued use of stimulants. Like Jacob and Justin, many people of all ages and walks of life battle with the seemingly invincible problem of stimulant addiction on a daily basis.

Does the scenario of Jacob or Justin describe you or someone you love? Are you searching for answers? There are millions of people just like you or someone you know who are desperately seeking for their way out. Like Jacob and Justin, many have found that way out. They were introduced to "the Way," the Lord Jesus Christ, and have joined thousands of addicts who have found freedom through this program called **Reformers Unanimous (RU)**. RU directs people to the Truth Who makes free. I speak of the Truth named the Lord Jesus Christ. Many have come to an RU meeting, facing a combination of destructive circumstances. Many have sought help on their own, like Jacob and Justin, without any long-term success. Yet, these same people are transformed as they engage in the RU curriculum and participate in its extremely supportive weekly programs.

Thousands of these individuals are now productive members of society. Collectively, they are a living testimony that there is hope for you or for those whom you love.

Yes, stimulants CAN be eliminated from your life. There is hope! There is freedom! And, that is the gospel TRUTH!

UPPERS
THE TOPIC

Each stimulant user knows exactly how stimulants make them feel. They also recognize that the feeling it generates each time is fairly consistent. However, very few stimulant users actually know why it makes them feel this way, much less how it happens.

As with all other addictive drugs, it is amazing to learn how effective they are at masking the real root problem in a person's life. Stimulants actually manipulate neurotransmitters in the brain that create a false sense of well being. This sense of pleasure and calmness is, of course, only temporary. As well, it is not reality. However, we have a very great Creator who made our body to secrete these neurotransmitters, and He has ways of doing so without the pain and misery of stimulant abuse.

NEUROTRANSMITTERS AND THEIR ROLES IN THE BODY:

- Acetylcholine: stimulates muscles, aids in sleep cycle
- Norepinephrine: similar to adrenaline, increases heart rate; helps form memories
- GABA (gamma-aminobutyric acid): prevents anxiety
- Glutamate: aids in memory formation
- Serotonin: regulates mood and emotion
- Endorphin: necessary for pleasure and pain reduction
- Dopamine: motivation; pleasure

In this chapter, Dr. George Crabb, a board certified Internal Medicine physician and member of the American Society of Addiction Medicine, will explain to us the phenomenon and feeling of this mood and mind-altering drug of choice for so many.

Jacob, who we read about earlier, experienced the effects of a chemical known as *methylphenidate*. This chemical is also known as Ritalin and Concerta. Justin experienced the effects of the chemical *amphetamine*, also known as Adderall. We generally know this class of medications as stimulants. Stimulants are one of world's most powerful drugs abused by thousands. To understand the effects of stimulants on Jacob and Justin, we will first look at how these chemicals worked on their brains.

Ritalin, Adderall, and the other stimulants stimulate the central nervous system by effecting the release and uptake of dopamine, which is one of the naturally-occurring neurotransmitters in our brains. These stimulants work to block the re-uptake of the neurotransmitter dopamine, making more of it available in the brain. The dopamine stimulates the brain's frontal lobes, limbic system, and cortex, thereby activating the brain's behavior control center. The frontal lobes are responsible for concentration, decision making, planning, learning, and retention. Like many medications, these stimulants have many short term and long term side effects.

STIMULANT FACT

Ritalin was first synthesized in 1944 in an attempt to find an effective treatment for depression, chronic fatigue syndrome, and narcolepsy.

SHORT-TERM SIDE EFFECTS:

- Nervousness
- Heart Palpitations
- Insomnia
- Headaches
- Loss of Appetite
- Arrhythmias
- Nausea and Vomiting
- Increased Blood Pressure
- Dizziness
- Skin Rashes and Itching
- Abdominal Pain
- Weight Loss
- Digestive Problems
- Psychotic Episodes

NOTE: *In rare cases, toxic psychosis may develop. An individual may experience depression when stopping the medication.*

LONG-TERM SIDE EFFECTS:

- Loss of Appetite
- Anxiety
- Tremors and Muscle Twitching
- Restlessness

- Fever
- Paranoia
- Convulsions
- Hallucinations
- Headaches (Severe Migraines)
- Delusions
- Arrhythmias
- Excessive Repetition of Movements
- Respiratory Problems
- Meaningless Task and Formication

Jacob was one of many people who was using Ritalin for non-medical purposes. He was taking the medicine only for the feeling, the "high" that results from taking it.

According to the 2005 Monitoring the Future Survey (MTF) conducted among United States' students, 2.4 percent of students in eighth grade have abused Ritalin in the past year. Tenth grade students represent 3.4 percent and 4.4 percent of twelfth graders. Studies have also indicated that non-medical use of Ritalin, Adderall, and other stimulants occur mostly in boys, but there has been an increasing trend noted in girls. This increasing trend has thought to be related not only to the high achieved with this medication but also to the weight loss results because the medication suppresses a person's appetite.

How did a drug meant to help become a favorite recreational drug? The non-medical use of prescription medications has become an enormous problem in North America in the past few years. Our younger generation is looking for an "edge." They have found this so-called edge in Ritalin and other stimulants. Ritalin as well as Adderall are stimulants and give the abuser a high. The medication "kick starts" the user's ability to focus and concentrate long after others with his or her schedule would have gone to bed. The ability to stay ahead of others is a reason cited by many as the reason they begin using Ritalin or Adderall. This is a highly-competitive world and to get ahead, which is the goal of many people, requires long hours and lots of hard work. Many feel they need to use a stimulant in order to do well. Many are not satisfied with their natural abilities. They have a sense of inadequacy or pressure that is often carried throughout life that is temporarily relieved by the use of stimulants.

According to John Hopkins University's 2002 newsletter, more than seven million children in the United States take an estimated eight tons of Ritalin every year. One of the major reasons why Ritalin has become so abused is its availability. With more prescriptions being written, there are more potential sources of the medication for people without prescriptions. According to the DEA, most Ritalin intended for abuse comes from legitimately-obtained supplies.

Physician shopping (the practice of going to different doctors to obtain prescriptions) is another way of getting Ritalin. I have had these people come to my office on many occasions, and it is amazing what stories they tell me in order to get their prescription. Ritalin is usually taken in its easiest and simplest form as a pill. However, people can inject the drug directly into their veins, or they can also crush the drug and snort the drug nasally.

Some people have told me that Ritalin is prescribed to millions of children in the United States alone, and they go on to comment that it is prescribed by a health care professional and approved by the FDA, so how harmful can it be? These comments are a sample of the faulty logic that many Ritalin and Adderall abusers use when discussing the safety of their drug of choice. Yes, millions of children do take Ritalin! Yes, it is prescribed by health care professionals! Yes, it is FDA approved! But, that does not mean it will not cause harm when taken in ways other than prescribed. Drug abuse and the drug problem are not limited to the selling and using of drugs such as cocaine or heroin (or even steroids), but the biggest drug problem today is the abuse of prescription medications. The non-medical use of prescriptions drugs has increased dramatically. According to the NSDUA, in 2002, an estimated 4.7 million Americans used prescription drugs for non-medical purposes for the first time.

The risk of abusing Ritalin and other methylphenidates, as well as Adderall and other forms of amphetamines, comes from how the drugs are abused as well as the characteristics of the drugs themselves. The person who injects the medication runs the risk of contracting HIV, Hepatitis B, or even Hepatitis C when they share needles. More common are complications caused by the pills' fillers, which do not dissolve in water. When the solution is injected, these particles can block tiny blood vessels causing damage to the lungs and even to the eyes. If the powder of a crushed pill is inhaled, nasal passages can become irritated, and in some cases, lung damage has been reported. People who abuse Ritalin, Adderall, or other prescription medications are lured into a false sense of security simply by the fact that these drugs require a prescription by a physician or other health care professionals. However, this does NOT make them safe!

Jacob and Justin, as they would take Ritalin and Adderall, felt more energetic or more "raring to go." These are some of the things that make taking these types of medications attractive to overworked and frustrated young people as well as those looking for more party ability.

These stimulants can affect blood pressure and cause the heart to beat irregularly or too fast. Blood pressure can increase so dramatically that the individual may suffer a stroke. A change in the person's heart rhythm can cause a heart attack, even in a child or teenager. Although the physical side effects of these types of medication are fairly well known, that is not true of the psychiatric reactions to their abuse. Psychiatric side effects that have been reported resemble ones that are associated with methamphetamine and cocaine abuse. Some of the psychiatric side effects of these stimulants are:

- Extreme Anger with Threats of Violence
- Delirium
- Severe Panic Attacks

Ritalin and Adderall dependency and addiction can be characterized by the need for increasingly higher doses of the drug and increasingly frequent binges. Between binges, those abusing the drug often fall into deep depression. The only way out of that depression is more of the medication. Ritalin, Adderall, and other stimulants caused biological changes in the brains of Jacob and Justin. Because of these biological changes, stimulant withdrawal is a very serious issue. As they withdrew from these stimulants, they experienced some of the following:

- Severe Agitation
- Sleeplessness
- Abdominal Cramps
- Nausea
- Depression
- Exhaustion
- Anxiety

Ask Jacob or Justin or anyone else who has withdrew from these types of stimulants about the effects. They will, without exception, describe a nightmare.

Before closing this chapter on stimulants, I want to discuss briefly an over-the-counter stimulant that is highly abused by many. This chemical is called *ephedra*. Ephedra and *ephedrine* containing dietary supplements have proven to be among the most dangerous of all over-the-counter stimulants. These products include:

- ma huang
- Chinese ephedra
- Sida
- cordifolia

Ephedrine-containing products and Xendrine are advertised to approve athletic performance and to dramatically increase weight loss. Structurally, there is not much difference between ephedrine and amphetamines, like Ritalin and Adderall. Ephedrine stimulates the central nervous system (brain and spinal cord) and works as a decongestant. Though it is an effective treatment for certain sinus and bronchial symptoms, it can cause a dangerous tachycardia, and it can also increase blood pressure. Heart attacks, strokes, intracranial bleeding, and death have been associated with the misuse of these chemicals. Marketing ploys have indicated that ephedrine-containing supplements are good alternatives to illegal street drugs, such as Ecstasy. The FDA has advised people to stay away from any supplement making those claims. Ephedrine side effects include:

- Heart Attack
- Dizziness
- Stroke
- Gastrointestinal Distress
- Seizures
- Heart Palpitations
- Psychosis
- Irregular Heart Beat (including Tachycardia)
- Headache
- Potential Death

Friend, regardless of where you may be in your struggle with stimulant (Ritalin, Adderall, etc.) addiction, the good news is that there is life after stimulants. Jacob and Justin found this life. For this to be accomplished in your life, there must be a change in your behavior. I want you to know that the only effective way of changing your behavior is changing the beliefs to which you hold. This will be the subject of the remainder of this book.

WEED

WEED
THE TESTIMONIES

Steve's Testimony

I first experimented with marijuana in my high school years, but because I feared the effects of marijuana, I mostly drank alcohol. I know that sounds crazy, but that is the way a thirteen year old boy thinks. I began smoking marijuana in my thirties, a little bit before my marriage. At first I would only smoke other people's pot when it was introduced at a party or over at a friend's house. The friends that I was hanging with were a big factor initially as I developed an appetite for my drug of choice – marijuana. I found myself hanging out more and more with the friends who could supply me with my new addiction. I enjoyed the sensation of being high and the illusion of confidence it gave me. After a while, I learned how to mask any signs that I was doing the drug.

One good friend with whom I had been close to since high school made it easy for me to get high whenever I wanted to. He always had a generous supply for himself and sold the drug also. He was known for always getting high by all of our mutual friends, and he clearly had a problem. I didn't, of course! Eventually, I wanted to have my own supply so I could get high on my own. I began purchasing marijuana from him in bulk. This would last me a few weeks at a time, enough for me to smoke everyday. Not wanting to grow too dependent on my old friend as my only source, I also began purchasing it from people at work. I was vaguely aware that my actions were beginning to become dangerous, at least as far as threatening my job if I were caught. This, however, was not enough to hinder me. I began to take foolish chances. I knew that my job had no drug screening policy, and it was easy to find people that would sell it to me. I would wait until after work and make the exchange in the parking lot. I would roll one up and smoke it on the way home. It was not long until I had a few friends who wanted to buy the drug from me. I, of course, readily complied. My wife would caution me that I could now be considered a dealer if I kept this up. She said my name would appear in the paper, and I would be stigmatized for the rest of my life. This made me a little concerned but nothing that getting high could not make me forget.

As months and years passed, I began to see how getting high every night made me more apathetic to the real world. I had goals and dreams that didn't seem to matter any more. If I was troubled about this during the sober times of the day, I could forget about it when I got high. I did not need to deal with anything important nor did I want to. There were those sober times when I would remember, and it would nag at me. Once in a while, I would vow to cut down and not do it every night, just on the weekends. But, by this time, I was hooked! It owned me, and I could not stop nor decrease my intake for any length of time. No amount of my own willpower was going to help me. The more trapped I felt by my addiction, the more I would get high to forget. It was a vicious cycle, and I was powerless to overcome it. I now began smoking pot in front of friends that did not approve of my new lifestyle. I remember seeing the disappointment on their faces. At no time would any of these friends try to get me to stop. They would just kid with me about it.

Something, however, happened that changed everything! In the fog of my years of smoking dope, I began to remember my desire to have a family with children. I spoke to my wife about it, and she said that it would not be possible unless we stop smoking pot and start going to church. My wife and I were raised Catholic, but something happened to my wife somewhere along the way. Thus, she insisted on going to a Baptist church. Not being a big fan of my former church, I went along with her. After going to a few churches that my wife did not seem satisfied with for some mysterious reason, we came upon a Baptist church just a few miles from our home. We both loved it! The pastor and people were very friendly, and I could sense that there was something different about this church. We began attending the Sunday morning services. My wife warned me that this was a type of church that would come and visit us. Sure enough, the following Thursday evening there was knock on the door. We were in the basement getting high so we did not answer the door. Something, though, impressed me about a church that would come and visit you at your home. This never happened in my previous church. "Did this church really care about us?" I wondered. The next Thursday night there was another knock at the door. I did not know whether to be happy or annoyed. Again, we did not answer, but we did keep returning to the church services. I would listen intently to the preaching. I kept hearing the pastor speak about getting saved and how we must all be born again. I asked my wife about it but was not ready to relinquish my sin.

Then, one day we got a call on our answering machine. It was the church's secretary. She wanted to know if it was okay if the pastor and his wife stopped by for a visit the following Thursday. I thought to myself, "Is she serious!" "The pastor and his wife want to come and see us?" How could I say no! In all of my years going to my former church, no one ever paid me a visit. To say I was nervous was an understatement. I was trying to quit marijuana at this time, but the thought of having the pastor over drove me to chain smoking. Attending the church services was one thing but having the pastor and his wife in my home was another. When the pastor arrived at my house on Thursday night, I was so nervous. My wife began chatting with them about her salvation experience and how God had been dealing with her to get right. I felt a little relieved because no one was really paying attention to me. No sooner had I had this thought when my wife turned to me and said, "Steve, do you have something to tell the pastor?" What was on my heart just flooded out of my mouth, and I declared, "I am not saved!" That night, that man of God, and now my pastor, led me to the Lord. I accepted Jesus Christ as my Savior, and I was born again that very minute. I was beaming with a joy I had never known before, and I was excited to know that the Holy Spirit was now living inside of me. The following week I was baptized and added to the church. This same church had a program that I had been hearing about during the announcements. This program is called Reformers Unanimous. My sister-in-law, Mary, who was visiting us at the time, told us that she attended a Reformers Unanimous program in Syracuse, New York and highly recommended the program to my wife and me. It was not long before we were approached by the RU director at our church to get involved. This man's enthusiasm was infectious, and his love for the Lord was obvious. He told me how vital it was to have a personal relationship with my new Savior and that Reformers Unanimous would help me develop one. I decided to give it a try. It has been two and a half years, and I have not looked back once! Not only do I consider my RU director and his wife among my dearest and closest friends, but I am involved in a ministry helping others off of their addictions and introducing them to my Savior as well. My second-talk group is always a source of encouragement as we support and pray for each other.

The Lord, Jesus Christ, has been so good to my wife and me. We left behind the chains of our bondage of marijuana. We now have a new addiction to serving and loving our Savior! I am now a bus captain and bring in about fifty kids a week to church, some of who attend the Reformers Unanimous Children's Program. We are also able to offer the Reformers Unanimous Program to the bus children's parents, many of whom are addicted to drugs. Now, when we knock on doors, we are known as the "church people." At first, they think we are a couple of "goody two shoes." However, when we share with them, they see that we are just like them. And, we know SOMEONE who can help them, too. Not long after I was saved, I was doing my Saturday morning bus visiting, and as I approached the home of one of my bus kids, I glanced down and something caught my eye. There in the gutter was a pretty large marijuana cigarette. I had to smile as I looked up to Heaven, and I thanked my God that I no longer wanted anything like that in my life. What a privilege it is to have a purpose for my life and a harvest field to work in for the Savior who made me free.

Steve could not take the internal pain any longer. He saw no way to escape the pain or sense of hopelessness except through continued use of marijuana. Like Steve, many people of all ages and walks of life battle with the seemingly invincible problem of marijuana addiction on a daily basis.

Does the scenario of Steve describe you or someone you love? Are you searching for answers? There are millions of people just like you or someone you know who are desperately seeking for their way out. Like Steve, many have found that way out. They were introduced to "the Way," the Lord Jesus Christ, and have joined thousands of addicts who have found freedom through this program called **Reformers Unanimous (RU)**. RU directs people to the Truth Who makes free. I speak of the Truth named the Lord Jesus Christ. Many have come to an RU meeting, facing a combination of destructive circumstances. Many have sought help on their own, like Steve, without any long-term success. Yet, these same people are transformed as they engage in the RU curriculum and participate in its extremely supportive weekly programs.

Thousands of these individuals are now productive members of society. Collectively, they are a living testimony that there is hope for you or for those whom you love. Yes, marijuana CAN be eliminated from your life. There is hope! There is freedom! And, that is the gospel TRUTH!

WEED
The Topic

Each marijuana user knows exactly how marijuana makes them feel. They also recognize that the feeling it generates each time is fairly consistent. However, very few marijuana users actually know why it makes them feel this way, much less how it happens.

As with all other addictive drugs, it is amazing to learn how effective they are at masking the real root problem in a person's life. Marijuana actually manipulates neurotransmitters in the brain that create a false sense of well being. This sense of pleasure and calmness is, of course, only temporary. As well, it is not reality. However, we have a very great Creator who made our body to secrete these neurotransmitters, and He has ways of doing so without the pain and misery of marijuana abuse.

NEUROTRANSMITTERS AND THEIR ROLES IN THE BODY:

- Acetylcholine: stimulates muscles, aids in sleep cycle
- Norepinephrine: similar to adrenaline, increases heart rate; helps form memories
- GABA (gamma-aminobutyric acid): prevents anxiety
- Glutamate: aids in memory formation
- Serotonin: regulates mood and emotion
- Endorphin: necessary for pleasure and pain reduction
- Dopamine: motivation; pleasure

In this chapter, Dr. George Crabb, a board certified Internal Medicine physician and member of the American Society of Addiction Medicine, will explain to us the phenomenon and feeling of this mood and mind-altering drug of choice for so many.

Steve, who we read about earlier, experienced the effects of the chemical, marijuana, found in the plant, *Cannibis Sativa*. Marijuana, also known as "Cannibis" or "hemp," is dried parts of the plant, everything from the leaves to the flowers and seeds, are used as a hallucinogen. Steve told us that he liked the feeling that marijuana gave him. He went on to tell me that marijuana put him in another state of mind. He felt relaxed. It appeared that all of his problems were disappearing, but as Steve now knows, his problems were not disappearing but getting worse because the good feelings marijuana gave him came at a significant price.

Marijuana, for the most part, is considered by its users as a "relatively mild drug." However, marijuana, as Steve found out, can lead to serious consequences just like any other drug. In fact, marijuana is dangerous and addictive, and it is known as one of the "gateway" drugs along with alcohol that generally opens the gate or door for the user to advance to more "hard core" drugs.

In 1970, the Controlled Substances Act was passed. This law classified marijuana, along with drugs like LSD and heroin, as a schedule I drug, meaning it had a high-risk of abuse and no acceptable medicinal use.

Steve has since found out that marijuana, like cigarettes and many other addictive drugs, does not contain just one single chemical. While more than 400 different substances can be found in one joint, the most common chemical is *delta-nine-tetrahydrocannabinol* or THC. The amount of THC determines how strong the marijuana is. The more THC in the drug, the more potent it is. As drug dealers and the drug culture have intensified, the marijuana smoked thirty years ago was less powerful than what is smoked today. This does give the users, like Steve, a stronger high but also subjects them to more harmful consequences.

Steve generally smoked his marijuana in the form of a joint. A *joint* is a hand-rolled cigarette containing marijuana. A hand-rolled cigar containing marijuana is called *blunts*. Blunts often contain other drugs as well as marijuana, with the most common additive being crack cocaine.

When Steve inhaled the marijuana smoke, the THC was taken into his body, and the fat in his body organs absorbed the chemical. The drug's smoke acts in a similar way to tobacco smoke, passing through the lungs and into the blood stream. From there, it is carried to the organs, with the most important of these being the brain. As the THC entered Steve's brain, the chemical would connect to specific receptors on the nerve cells. These receptors are known as *cannabinoid* receptors. These receptors allow the THC to affect the activities of the cells to which it binds. The majority of the drug's effects are felt in the areas of the brain that control the following:

1. Memory

2. Concentration
3. Thought
4. Pleasurable Feelings
5. Perception of Time – Senses – Movements

Marijuana's ability to impair performance and dramatically increase the heart rate is related to the concentration of THC in the batch of marijuana. This is a variable amount, so users like Steve may not always be able to predict the effects marijuana will have on them. As mentioned earlier, the smoke of a marijuana joint can contain hundreds of chemicals. Steve has come to find out that marijuana smoke can be just as harmful as tobacco smoke, as it contains similar amounts of such harmful compounds as:

• Carbon monoxide
• Hydrogen cyanide
• Tar

NOTE: Smoking marijuana increases your risk of developing cancer!

In light of the above, marijuana is one of the most commonly-used illicit drugs in the United States. More than forty percent of people over the age of twelve have tried the drug at least once. In 2002, marijuana was the cause of more than 119,000 emergency room visits. This made it the third most prevalent abused drug. This is a huge problem for our young people, for we understand by Steve's testimony that he was introduced to marijuana at the young age of thirteen. A recent survey indicated that sixteen percent of eighth graders have tried marijuana. The percentage dramatically increases for tenth graders at thirty-five percent, as well as a significant increase for twelfth graders at forty-six percent. In light of this, it was noted by the National Household Survey on Drug Abuse that marijuana was the most widely used drug among teenagers. Many young people, like Steve, started using marijuana for many reasons. A very common reason is peer pressure. The young person feels that they will be isolated or not accepted if they don't participate. Also, many young people have told me in the privacy of my office that they use marijuana as an escape from problems and stress at home and school. Steve went on to tell me that, to an extent, he used marijuana to rebel against his parents. Upon further questioning, he stated that by using marijuana, he was demonstrating or proving to others that he could be independent. To Steve, marijuana was a reminder of how he could make his own decisions and take care of himself. But, most go back to using marijuana for the simple reason that it serves as a release, albeit temporary, from their problems.

The person could be a user because of:

- A Troubled Home Environment
- An Unfulfilling Job
- Social Problems at School

Life's problems make people, like Steve, more likely to turn to marijuana. Some people use marijuana to escape from their inner torment, such as:

- Depression
- Feelings of Failure
- Feelings of Helplessness

People searching for a release from these feelings may think the solution lies in marijuana. Many individuals that use marijuana believe it is harmless, but it can cause serious health and mental problems. There are many possible responses to a drug like marijuana. When Steve would smoke marijuana, he generally felt a high, which he describes as feeling relaxed and happy. At times, he would have an increase in hunger or thirst. This is often known as the "munchies." But, there are more adverse effects of marijuana as well. And, as Steve probes into the many years of his addiction, these adverse effects were a part of his life. Marijuana increased anxiety in his life as well as a heightened sense of paranoia. While some of these effects are only temporary or short-lived, some can be permanent, including disruptions in perception, memory, and judgment. In fact, these long-term effects can last up to six weeks after the drug is used. I have also seen a condition in the emergency room known as *cannabis intoxication.* This is characterized by the following symptoms:

- Loss of Motor Coordination
- Loss of Judgment
- Anxiety
- Withdrawal
- Hallucinations

Marijuana also caused Steve's heart rate to increase, his eyes to become blood-shot, and also caused him to have a dry mouth. Now, while all of these side effects that I have described sound bad enough, others are more serious and have long-term consequences. Marijuana can disrupt your immune system. Marijuana kills the protective cells at the upper part of your airway, which makes it easier for germs to get into your body and cause damage. Marijuana also reduces the body's ability to fight off harmful diseases. This means that people who smoke marijuana are more likely to die from an otherwise treatable disease like pneumonia, which often proves fatal in people with weakened immune systems even though we have more advanced medicine and technology in our world today. As Steve smoked marijuana, it killed helpful cells in his body like *macrophages* and *T-cells*, which are responsible for fighting off germs in the body. When these are gone, disease can overtake a person's body very easily. Smoking marijuana increases the chance of getting cancer in the head or neck. Marijuana, in fact, may be more of a cancer threat than tobacco as it contains four times the amount of tar that one regular cigarette does. Marijuana users are putting themselves at an even greater risk of developing cancer than tobacco users. Smoking marijuana not only increases your chance of developing lung cancer but also increases your risk of developing diseases such as emphysema and chronic bronchitis. A recent study that I came across stated that those who use marijuana frequently have more health problems. They feel sick more and miss more days of work and school than those who do not smoke marijuana. Smoking marijuana increases the chance of a heart attack in as much as four times more than in an individual that does not smoke this drug. It increases blood pressure and heart rate. It also causes the blood to lose some of its ability to carry oxygen, making the heart work much harder.

As we have discussed the many problems that marijuana can cause to various body organs, the brain is the organ that is most adversely affected. Marijuana users are more prone to panic attacks, flashbacks, delusions, paranoia, and hallucinations. First-time users can suffer from these results. This is all caused by the binding of THC to the various brain cells, many which are located in the brain that control memory, thought, and concentration. These nerve cells are influenced by the binding of THC to their receptors, and it also changes the concentration of the neurotransmitter *dopamine*, which regulates the feelings of motivation and pleasure. Marijuana can not only cause an increase in panic attacks and anxiety but also can cause depression. Steve suffered from both anxiety and depression, and these began to cause disruptions in his daily life. He started having difficulties learning new skills and remembering information, which ultimately led to him falling behind in work and other everyday responsibilities.

Like so many other drugs, marijuana can also have an adverse effect on unborn babies. Those mothers using marijuana during their pregnancy have an increased risk of miscarriages. Infants born to mothers using marijuana are often born premature or have low birth weights. These children have been noted to be more nervous and more apt to cry as well as having a different response to visual stimuli than most infants their age. This all points to a potential neurological defect in the baby's brain which was caused by the mother's marijuana use. As these children are followed from their birth into their elementary and secondary educational programs, they are found to have a higher frequency of abnormal behavior as well as poor academic performance.

Our society today is relatively alert to those who are driving under the influence of alcohol, but driving under the influence of marijuana is just as dangerous. Steve can tell you that the many times he drove under the influence of marijuana, his reaction time was delayed, he had a diminished ability to concentrate, and his coordination skills were diminished. He told me that he had a harder time responding to signals on the road, which led to many close calls as he drove. You see, marijuana impairs these necessary skills for at least four to six hours after using one joint, well after the user has lost the euphoria of the high. Marijuana is still just as addictive as any other drug that is out there. People will start to crave the drug and can not function without it. Steve made this most vivid in his testimony. He had an uncontrollable urge for the drug. He used the drug even when he knew the drug was not in his best interest. Steve, over time, developed a tolerance for the drug, which required more and more of it to give him the high he desired. During his active addiction, he was unable to cut down or control his use. He also had to start setting aside huge amounts of time to smoke the marijuana. He started to isolate himself, thus, decreasing his social activities because marijuana use was consuming more and more of his time. Even though down deep he understood the potential ramifications of his drug use, he continued to use. Steve was always thinking about it and thinking about when he could get his next high. He thought of marijuana as his friend, the cure for ALL of his problems. When Steve finally broke the bondage of marijuana addiction through Jesus Christ, his body experienced irritability, insomnia, and anxiety, which are all signs of marijuana withdrawal. For you see, the physical and mental aspect of who we are becomes dependent on the drug, and one finds it hard to survive without it. Steve also experienced tension headaches and a decreased appetite. While some of these symptoms appear within twenty-four hours of the last dose of marijuana, they can last up to twenty-eight days. Marijuana stays in the body long after the drug is consumed. Steve's body, especially the fat cells, absorbed the THC and transformed it into *metabolites* so the body can rid itself of this foreign, harmful substance. These *metabolites* can be found in the urine for up to a week after use.

Clearly, marijuana use has serious consequences associated with it. And, in fact, very few adolescents use other illicit drugs without first trying marijuana.

Friend, regardless of where you may be in your struggle with marijuana addiction, the good news is that there is life after marijuana. Steve found this life. For this to be accomplished in your life, there must be a change in your behavior. I want you to know that the only effective way of changing your behavior is changing the beliefs to which you hold. This will be the subject of the remainder of this book.

THE TRUTH

THE TRUTH

When viewing the world of addiction, we often envision a scenario of total victimization. But, the cold reality of addiction is that it is a deliberate, destructive choice made by the user that is followed by many other, similar bad choices. In other words, it is a lifestyle of repetitive, bad choices.

This "choice" is a release for the user, albeit, temporary. It relieves the pain that dwells in the deepest, darkest dungeon of one's life. A user may be thinking, "It is no big deal!" Choosing to believe that is merely one's attempt to minimize and deflect attention away from their problem. My friend, addiction is a big deal. It is a major issue that affects the body, soul, and spirit of an individual. You may think it is a necessary ingredient for having a good time or getting your work done, but oh how far from the truth is that lie?!

However, if you picked up this book at an RU class or received it in some way from someone who cares about you, then you might by thinking, "I know someone like that!" Or, you may even say, "That's me!"

So, why do you do what you do? The reasons behind your destructive behavior are many. Perhaps the most common reason for addiction is because it is a coping mechanism.

All of us learn to handle stressful and negative events in different ways. We feel "out of control" because of internal pain, frustration, and anxiety. Our natural response is to alleviate the pain. Unfortunately, many people find temporary relief in the addiction of their choice.

Dr. Crabb is 100 percent correct. If you find yourself living your life this way, then you have developed an unhealthy coping mechanism. A coping mechanism is simply how a person chooses to deal with disappointments. Prior to my role as Reformers Unanimous President and Founder, I was addicted to marijuana, powder cocaine and alcohol for over ten years. Whenever I would use marijuana, cocaine or alcohol, the overwhelming difficulties from which I was running seemed to disappear.

I believe that our many inner hurts is what creates our desire to escape reality. That internal hurt drives one to use drugs or alcohol as a way to relieve the pain. But, unfortunately, the pain and hurt is always still there when the drugs or alcohol is gone.

As someone who personally knows the bondage of marijuana, cocaine, and alcohol and has found freedom from their gripping control, I want you to know that believing your hard or hurt feelings are best handled with the coping mechanisms of methamphetamine, marijuana, cocaine, alcohol, or another mood altering drug is an absolute lie. It is a lie from your spiritual enemy, Satan, who seeks to entrap then destroy you. Our desire is to reveal to you the Truth. If you will choose to reject any lies you have believed and choose to live in this Truth you are learning, then the power the lies possess over you will be broken. The Bible promises those who Jesus has made free are freed indeed (see John 8:36 at the back of this book for actual Bible wording)!

This "choice" is only a temporary fix. It does not remove the pain caused by your unmet needs. It simply temporarily masks it. The condemnation and feelings of guilt and shame that many addicts carry from past failures, abuses, or unhealthy relationships inside and outside the family can lead to a self-hatred deep in their soul for which they desperately desire relief.

You have chosen a coping mechanism, choosing it to be your preferred way of dealing with this internal turmoil. This improperly handled internal turmoil eventually leads the user to become depressed. Depression then facilitates increased use. Always remember this: Depression can and usually will control your entire life.

Feelings of depression lead a person to feel that they have no control and that things will never change. They feel they are in a deep, dark hole with no legitimate way out. They see the only way out to escape their mental anguish is take a break from reality. Depression coupled with even occasional drug use can be a life-threatening combination.

An addict's thinking is all based on a lie. Having accepted this lie, they now have a distorted view of reality. Their whole concept of life has become skewed. How could someone come to believe that something so damaging and destructive can bring relief? The answer is found in this truth: Wrong behavior is stimulated by a process of wrong thinking. Wrong thinking is permeated by wrong beliefs.

To change our behavior, we must change our thinking. And, to change our thinking, we will need to change a great many of our wrong beliefs about ourselves, God, and even about others. In other words, our beliefs must be dealt with in order to experience eventual, true and lasting freedom.

So, we see that addiction is a vicious cycle with no apparent way out. However, there is a way of escape! I have escaped and am no longer an addict. You have tried to find your own way of escape, haven't you? It has not happened. You have constantly failed. Your failures have only increased your addiction and its hold on your life, leading to deeper pain. But, the Bible has the answer.

Jesus, whom in John 8:32 tells us is "the Truth," beckons for you to turn to Him. He wants to break the chains that hold you in bondage. He wants to restore and comfort you into a right relationship to God, to others, and even to ourselves.

Dr. Crabb is an expert on addiction recovery. As a member of the American Society of Addiction Medicine, he has partnered with me and our ministry to help everyone understand that the real bondage of addiction is not physical, or even mental. It is spiritual.

The Truth of Jesus and the truths of Jesus will give you a life of joy. Jesus called it an "abundant life." But, how do you find Him? And, how do you find the submission to Him necessary to be made free?

Those are good questions. Allow me to introduce to you the Answer, Jesus Christ. He is the answer that I have found in my quest to be cured of marijuana, cocaine, and alcohol addiction. Jesus is the only One who can touch your heart so deeply that your life can literally change forever.

Our media tends to portray Christians in a very unattractive way. They even like to make them look stupid or "extra dependant" on a crutch of some sort to get through life. I've heard it said on national television by a well known actor that "Christians are weak people who can't stand the thought that they only have one life, so live it up! They just gotta' believe in giving this life up for some hope of another world that doesn't exist!"

Can I ask a question? How would a Hollywood actor know if there is another world? And, if he is wrong and I am right, how sorry would he be that he was on the wrong end of that opinion.

It is sad that Christians are portrayed on television and in movies as idiots because this portrayal has a profound impact on those who are so gullible to society's ways of manipulation. The truth is that very smart people, many presidents, kings, mega large corporate CEO's, and millions of others profess themselves to be believers in Jesus Christ as their only way to Heaven. Are they stupid, gullible, or in need of some crutch? I would say not.

As a matter of fact, you know what? They are happy people! A great many of them live victorious lives over vice. It is almost unheard of for a Christian to commit suicide. There must be a reason why so many rich or famous people who do not possess Christ profess such misery in life. They are unable to find any satisfaction though they have tried and tried and tried.

Yes, the world is influenced by Hollywood actors, media moguls and personalities, millions of other CEO's who are miserable; but there are even more engineers, machinists, construction workers, secretaries, wait-staff, and busy mothers who do not know this Christ of whom I speak. Glaringly, you can see their lifestyle bound to selfish pride, ingratitude, depression, and many other debilitating behaviors.

I think it is easier to believe in a Creator that put you here for a reason and wants you to be at peace with Him and to fulfill that reason for your existence than it is to believe, "We only live once—enjoy it!" Boy, I would hate to be wrong on that decision and live eternity in hell because I would rather continue in wrong and never be forgiven for it.

Jesus came to make us free. He will make you free from guilt, shame, condemnation, and hatred. He will make you free to enjoy a life of peace, joy, satisfaction, and among other things, sobriety. Jesus will illuminate the root causes of your addiction. Not only will He show you the problem, He will show you the answer to your problem. Jesus will never harm, hurt, or betray you. The love Jesus has for you will never change because His love is not based on you or your performance, but solely based on His character, which never, ever changes.

The Bible tells us that, to conform our lives to something worthwhile and fulfilling, we must transform the way that we think. (See Romans 12:2 in the back of this book.) Transformation is the word metamorphosis. It means "to change in form." In this case, we want to change our forms of thinking. The best way to change our way of thinking is not to "try" to think differently, but rather to first change the way we believe. When our beliefs change, then so can our thoughts.

For example, you remember the super hero the Incredible Hulk? Whenever his alter ego, David Bruce Banner, became angry or outraged, a startling "metamorphosis" occurred. He went from being calm, cool, and collected to a raging monster because he struggled to handle adversity. Anger was a trigger that changed this otherwise calmed man into the form of a monster. That was a negative and dangerous transformation.

However, there was another super hero that was far more "mild mannered." I am speaking of Clark Kent. Clark Kent never broke a sweat when faced with adversity. How could he stay so calm, so cool, and so collected no matter the level of threat he faced? It was because he knew he had a power living within him that gave him supernatural abilities. Clark Kent, remembering this during extremely difficult times, made it possible for himself to "transform" into a dependable person in times of trouble.

Well, that is the transformation we all need! And, that, my friend, is the transformation that RU wants you to experience. Not a transformation in which you become a super hero, but one in whom you become Supernatural.

There are three benefits of salvation (accepting the truth…JESUS): justification, sanctification, and glorification. It is these benefits that grant us not only the freedom from sin's penalty, but also the freedom from sin's power, and eventual freedom from sins' presence.

In our next chapter, we will explain to you how to have your payment for your sin debt (death and hell) paid by the One who died for all. We want everyone who attends our classes to clearly understand how they can accept Jesus Christ, the Truth, as their personal Savior. We will do this here for you by explaining to you God's Simple Plan of Justification. It comes from a complete transformation.

THE TRUTH
OUR TRANSFORMATION THROUGH JUSTIFICATION

Now, I understand that the purchase of this book indicates that you or someone you love struggles with some type of stubborn habit or possibly even an addiction. . And you probably were not necessarily interested in finding religion; you want to find FREEDOM! But, my friend, there is no freedom without the Son of God. If you want to be freed, you will have to go through the only Way that grants freedom. You gain freedom through the sacrifices made on our behalf by Jesus Christ.

Jesus wants to help you! He has already provided a way of escape for you. Choosing to continue in your behavior is, in essence, denying and rejecting the freedom Jesus offers to you. Trying to construct your own answers to your addiction or even your other problems in life is like saying that the torture Jesus went through for you on the cross was not enough. He would need to do more for you to turn to Him.

No! His death was enough to pay not only the penalty for your sin, but also to provide you with the emancipation from the power of your sin, as well. Yes, true freedom begins by accepting Jesus Christ's substitutionary death on the cross as your penalty payment for all the wrong you have ever committed. All of it, one payment. God's sinless Son died for you. We refer to this as "accepting Christ as your Savior."

If you have never done this in your life, there is no other step, much less twelve steps you can take to find freedom. This is a "change in belief" that each individual must make for themselves. It is the most important choice you will ever make.

Justification is a benefit that takes place at the moment of salvation. Justification is salvation from the *penalty* of sin (which is the Bible word for our wrongs). The penalty from which we are being justified is the penalty of eternal separation from God in a place called Hell.

To help you picture what Christ has done for you and me, there are some key words in the Bible I want to help you understand. What Jesus Christ actually did **for us** needs to be understood before we can clearly accept His gift and establish the pathway to freedom from our addictive nature.

SIN

Sin is the Bible word for our wrong. The Bible tells us that everyone does things wrong and everyone does wrong things. This makes us sinners. (See Romans 3:23)

Our wrongs must be paid for in some way and someday. It is a huge debt! The Bible tells us the payment for our wrong doing is death. (See Romans 6:23)

We are all sinners and so are you. Your drug of choice is just one of the many sin problems that you have. You may think the best choice you could make is avoid your stubborn habit or addictive behavior. But, the worst choice you can make is to die as an unconverted sinner. You will spend eternity in hell.

Do you really believe that you are a sinner? As you enter our program, ask yourself this question. "Do I realize I am a sinner, and that my sin deems me worthy of hell?" If you do not know this, your beliefs must change, my friend, if you are going to be made free in life.

Step One: Accept the fact that you are a sinner. Express to God in dependence upon Him your agreement with the Bible that you are indeed a wrong doer, a sinner!

DEATH

Death means to be absent of life. The Bible tells us that because of sin, God determined that man would become mortal. As a result of that decision, eventually each person physically dies because of our wrong doing. (See Romans 5:12)

However, if we die in our sins, we are destined for hell and separated from God for eternity. Hell is God's judgment and final rejection of the lost. But, it is not a rejection because of our imperfection; it is judgment for our rejection! God loves us, even as sinners, but our sin exempts us from our ability to enjoy Heaven (for those who do not accept His free gift of Salvation).

Our Transformation Through Justification | 208

That free gift was borne by God's Son, Jesus, who willingly offered His own life as a substitute to pay for our debt. Jesus paid our sin debt when He willingly submitted to die for us by being crucified on the cross. (See Romans 5:8)

Do you believe that Jesus died for you and me? If not, please remember that our beliefs must change, my friend, if we are going to be made free in life. Please don't die refusing to believe that you are a sinner and that Jesus died for you.

Step Two: As you continue your prayer from step one, agree with the Bible through your own personal dependence that Jesus died for your sins.

BURIAL

The Bible tells us that after Jesus died, His followers borrowed the tomb of a wealthy believer and laid Jesus' body to rest in that tomb. It was guarded every hour of the day by Roman soldiers. (See Matthew 27:62-65) After three whole days, some close friends of Jesus came to visit the tomb, and found it empty! The body of Jesus was missing! Some thought He had been stolen. But, the Bible says that an angel of the Lord was sitting nearby and informed Jesus' friends that He was gone, for He had risen from the dead. (See Matthew 28:5-7)

Do you believe that Jesus was buried for you? If not, please remember that our beliefs must change, my friend, if we are going to be made free in life. Please don't die refusing to believe that you are a sinner and that Jesus died and was buried for you.

Step Three: As you continue your prayer from step two, agree with the Bible through your own personal dependence that Jesus was buried and laid in state for three whole days.

RESURRECTION

Resurrection means "brought back to life. "The Bible tells us that God the Father raised Jesus, His Son, from the dead through the power of His Holy Spirit. (See First Peter 3:18.) Yes, after being crucified and lying in a tomb for three days, Jesus came out of the grave alive! Hundreds of eye witnesses saw Him, proving that this phenomenon is truth.

You see, God is love. God loved us so much that He sent His Son to die for us (See John 3:16.), and He loved His Son so much that He raised Him from the dead. You see, death's power over us would not have been conquered unless God could demonstrate His power over it. Thus, the resurrection of Jesus is important to understanding what He has done for us. Yes, God has power over life, and He has power over death. He can give us the *promise* of His life, and He can save us from our *penalty* of our death.

Do you believe that Jesus was resurrected from the dead by God through the power of His Holy Spirit? If not, please remember that our beliefs must change, my friend, if we are going to be made free in life. Please don't die refusing to believe that you are a sinner, that Jesus died, was buried, and rose from the dead the third day.

Step Four: As you continue your prayer from step three, agree with the Bible through your own personal dependence that you believe that Jesus rose from the dead after three days, by the empowering Holy Spirit.

These three simple words—death, burial, and resurrection—are three words that represent the miracle events that provide us freedom from the penalty of our sins. Receiving this payment frees us from paying the debt for our sin. If you have accepted this gift, then according to the Bible, you now have a home in heaven reserved for you. We do not get to heaven based on what we have done, but by believing in what Christ has done *for* us. We have to believe by dependence on the events described in these three words in order to be saved from Hell and granted a home in Heaven.

That brings us to our final two important word definitions. Those final two words are "believe" and "receive. "After this, we will focus on how depending on the events that surround these single word meanings will also help YOU overcome your addiction. These simple words, their meanings and the events we are defining will provide you, as it has us, a great peace that simple sobriety could never afford!

BELIEVE

The word **believe** means, "to be persuaded to accept a truth through complete dependency upon it." The Bible tells us that Jesus is the Truth and anyone who knows this Truth will be made free. (See John 14:6 and John 8:32)

However, in order for Jesus' sacrifice to be applied to our personal sin debt, we must "be persuaded to accept this Truth of Jesus' death, burial, and resurrection through complete dependency upon it. "When we are fully persuaded that something is true, we will depend upon that truth, that is to say, we will believe it!

Belief is another word for confidence or faith. But, your confidence in something must be accepted through a **complete dependence** upon the truth believed in order to qualify as real faith. In other words, in order to be saved, you must "completely depend on Jesus" as the payer of your sin debt through His DBR (death, burial, resurrection). We must have confidence in Him that leads us to depend on Him alone to save us from the debt we owe for our wrong doings in life.

With that said, we do not *need* to add good works, or join a church, or give money, or even "go to confession" to get to Heaven. We only depend on His DBR! That is what the Bible calls "saving faith. "We must **believe** *on* Him in order to **receive** Him. Now, what do we receive when we believe on Him?

RECEIVE

Receive means "to obtain from another. "The Bible tells us that if we will believe in our hearts that Jesus died on the cross and that God raised Him from the dead that we would be saved. (See Romans 10:9) When we are saved, our sin debt is paid and He gives to us eternal life. If you believe on Him, you will receive this from Him.

Eternal life is best defined as "life in perpetuity. "This is to say, it is a life that begins when we get saved (or, are born again) and lasts forever. That is why we can commit to you that your new life will provide you power over your addiction. It has for me and many others just like me.

Our eternal life cannot be taken from us. (See 1 John 5:1) It is a free gift that cannot be earned by doing good or be taken away by doing bad. It is yours, if you will only believe and receive. Should we? Oh, yes, we all should. Could we? Oh yes, we all could accept this free gift. But, would you? That is the most important question that you will ever answer.

Salvation also gives us the empowering of Internal Persuasion. When we receive Christ as our Savior, the Bible tells us that His Holy Spirit comes to live within us. (See Ezekiel 36:27.) He lives within our spirit in what the Bible calls our inner man. Within the inner man, your spirit and the

Spirit of God can have fellowship one with another. This is where we find our ability to worship God and the ability to gain victory over our vices, including all stubborn habits or addictions!

This is God's simple plan of salvation, benefit number one—justification. When we experience justification, we **have been saved** from the *penalty* of sin.

Would you like to believe and accept Jesus Christ as your Savior? It is the first step to freedom from the power of sin, but it is the most important step. This is the step that grants us the freedom we all need from the *penalty* of sin. As a matter of fact, if you find escape from any or all life crippling addictions yet die and go to hell, your sobriety will not have been worth it whatsoever.

Friend, I plead with you today to take this first step! Consider praying this simple prayer to God, meaning it from your heart. Saying this prayer is a way to declare to God that you are depending on Jesus Christ alone for your salvation. The words themselves will not save you. Only dependence (faith) on Jesus Christ can grant us our salvation!

PRAYER: "Father, I know that I am a sinner and my sins have separated me from you. I am truly wrong and deserve to be punished for it. But, do believe that your Son, Jesus Christ, died to pay my sin penalty. I believe that He was buried for three days and was resurrected from the dead by the power of the Holy Spirit. I believe Jesus is alive, and hears my prayers. I accept His payment for my sins and invite His Spirit to indwell me and empower me to overcome my wrong behaviors. In Jesus' name I pray, Amen."

If you have prayed this prayer, you need to let another Christian know as soon as possible. Contact your RU leader, your RU director, the church pastor, or another Christian friend so that they can help you fully understand each part of this decision.

Your belief systems are changing, and if you have placed your full dependence upon Jesus to give you salvation, you now have a Presence living within you that can give you the power to behave differently. In other words, now that you have changed just one of the ways you believed, you are now empowered to change the way you think. This simple step can forever change the way you act.

To overcome the world's many vices, this new relationship you have established with Jesus needs to be developed. This relationship is strengthened by the Power of the indwelling Holy Spirit. The more you know Jesus, not *about* Him, but the more you personally *know* Him, the more *freedom* you will experience over the wrong doings of which you have been forgiven. This personal relationship will set you, as it has us, on a pilgrimage toward the second benefit of your salvation, your sanctification.

THE TRUTH
OUR CONFORMATION THROUGH SANCTIFICATION

After we have experienced the transformation of justification, we can soon see a developing Power source within us that gives us the ability to behave differently. This Power source is the indwelling Holy Spirit of God. He is real, though it may seem spooky when defined. His Spirit gives us the ability to do things we would never be able to do in our own power. Not just overcoming our addictions, but living a life that is pleasing to God and man, loving your family and others, serving unselfishly and becoming a person who gives of oneself to meet the needs of others. These are just some of the great things that will be produced when you conform into the image of God.

The word **conform** means "to be poured into a mold." The world naturally pours its inhabitants into a mold. At this stage of your life, you are conformed to this world's belief system, which, by the way, got you in the trouble you are in. But, the Bible tells us that God does not want us conformed to this world, but rather He wants us conformed to the image of His Son Jesus Christ. (See Romans 12:2.) This takes place through a process that the Bible calls sanctification. Sanctification is the process whereby we actually develop a personal relationship with Jesus Christ, using the communication Tool of the indwelling Holy Spirit of God. At RU, we will help you understand not only the importance of this relationship, but also the simplicity of a dynamic love relationship with Jesus. At RU, our entire curriculum is designed to help you develop this relationship called sanctification.

Sanctification is the second of our three benefits in God's plan of salvation. Like justification, this takes place the moment we accept Jesus as our personal Savior. *Sanctification* means "to be set apart for sacred use." However, just because we are set apart for sacred use, does not mean that God is using all believers sacredly!

Many believers fail to disciple, or become students of Christ's. If we do not become students of Christ as disciples, we will never learn about Him. The information we will fail to gain will make it difficult for us to develop a relationship with Him. If we fail to enjoy the benefits of our sanctification, we will seldom enjoy the power of God on our lives!

Failing to develop a walk with Christ is the wrong way for a believer to live their new Christian life. If you make this mistake too, you will fail to overcome many different sins in your life, especially the addiction that brought you to our program.

At Reformers Unanimous, our program focus is on developing our students to enjoy the benefits of their sanctification. Our students consist of newborn believers and long-time believers that are discouraged and apathetic Christians. We help these students obtain their walk with God through our intense discipleship curriculum, effective and motivational classes, individual, personal and group counseling, navigational principles that lead to prosperity in life, and active participation in church related events. All of the personal development we invest in the students of RU is free of charge. The only charge at RU is for cost of the books you may *choose* to purchase.

During our class time, we are instructed to develop as our goals the following eight "ships" as our system for overcoming the power that our addictions have gained over us:

Worship—humbling oneself in order to exalt God in personal praise.

Discipleship—learning how God acts, how man acts, and how man acts when he is trying to act like God in his own power.

Relationship—developing intimacy through a daily talk with God that produces a day-long walk with God.

Fellowship—an association between people of like faith that we may enjoy the stability that comes from accountability.

Followship—placing our life's most important decisions and choices under the influence of our God-ordained leadership, our umbrella of protection.

Leadership—placing our time and talents under the jurisdictional oversight of our God-ordained leaders.

Stewardship—placing our tithe (to be explained later) where God demands and our treasures where God directs.

Apprenticeship—learning from a personal Spirit-filled trainer how to love God, love others, and to serve God and others out of an appreciation for that great love.

Each of these "ships" are developmental stages. They are detailed in the

Reformers Unanimous book, Eight Ships That Shape Your Ship—Shipshape! You can order this important book and many other RU materials at your chapter book table, church bookstore or online at www.reformu.com

In this spiritual booklet on addiction, it would be difficult to explain all that a believer needs to understand concerning the sanctification process. However, we will attempt to explain sanctification in this chapter as an overview of its many benefits to your new-found faith.

Please remember that sanctification is a lifelong process of aligning every part of your soul and body with the indwelling Spirit of the living God.

This DOES NOT take incredible work on our part. Rather, it takes an intimate walk where you and He seldom part!! This walk with the Christ that saved our soul will grant us the Power over any bad habit.

You see, when we first began to dabble with sinful vices, they did not bind us. They seldom even restricted us. They were enjoyable and satisfying in the many ways listed in chapter three. But, over the course of time, it began the process of becoming a stubborn habit. That stubborn habit is now a full-fledged addiction that is in the process of taking your whole world away from you. It was a four step process that placed you in this position.

Your addiction began as a **TOEHOLD**. As a toehold, it was a bit of an inconvenience at times, but did not really slow you down too much. The enjoyment was worth the nagging sensation you often felt the next day. However, as you fed that appetite, it only grew stronger. An appetite once fed never grows weaker. It only grows stronger.

Eventually this habit grew to be a **FOOTHOLD**. As a foothold, it slowed your progress. You didn't seem to advance as quickly or recover as fast from the mistakes this habit was causing you to make.

However, you still advanced, albeit awkwardly, and you still recovered. But, eventually, your foothold became a **STRONGHOLD**. As a stronghold, it has become, well, just that—something that has a strong hold on you. As a stronghold, it not only slows your progress, but it also slows your productivity, like a pair of handcuffs would. You are not as productive in your personal life or your professional life and everything begins to fall apart.

It is at this stage that most of our students reach out to our "out-patient" local church addictions program for help. They are still functioning in society, but barely. They are losing jobs, experiencing failed marriages and their homes are often broken at this stage. It is sad when they are at this point in their life for often they are just beginning to look for help. But, it is a very difficult process to find freedom on your own. I believe it is nearly impossible. Without Jesus you may find sobriety, but you will not find contentment in the difficult journey of life.

However, some reject the solutions that many programs offer them and carry on with their addictive habits until the addiction develops from a stronghold into a full blown **STRANGLEHOLD**. A stranglehold will takes us wherever it wants us to go and restricts us from going anywhere we may want to go. Though a stronghold will bind you, a stranglehold will enslave you. It will control your entire life's existence. You live to feed it, and if you don't feed it, you will begin to think you are going to die!
At the stranglehold stage, you are a non-functioning addict. At this point, you will probably need a full-time residential program. This is the stage we find most of our applicants to our men's and women's residential Schools of Discipleship homes in Rockford, IL. The folks in our homes are barely functioning and they CANNOT find freedom unless they leave behind their troubled environment.

Our residential Schools of Discipleship (www.ruhomes.org) is a program that acts like a green house. It protects an addict from their environment so that they can grow really fast. If this is where you find yourself, please understand that those whose addiction appears to have a stranglehold on them will find great help at RU and the church that hosts it, but it may be necessary to take a break for a period of months in your life and recover from the snare in which you have found yourself.

With these four stages of addiction understood, we can see how sanctification is not the only lifelong process. Your personal destruction has been developing for a great portion of your life, as well. The moment we begin to rebel as young men or women against the authority system that God designed, we began a journey that leads to our eventual ruin. For me, that ruin emanated from addictive, sinful habits that I formed as a young man in rebellion to my parent's wishes.

For most people with addiction problems, it has taken a long time to develop these bad habits. It will take some time as well until your spiritual development will be strong enough to overcome those habits. However, most of our students see great victory almost instantaneously and experience lasting victory shortly thereafter. Why? Because in the process of sanctification, it is God that does the work, not the recovering addict.

With that said, God intends for our recovery process to begin at conversion through the justification of our soul and the sanctification of our spirit. God intends for the benefits of sanctification to begin at our conversion to Christ and to be increasing in enjoyment throughout the remainder of our lifetime. In justification, we are "made right in heaven." Sanctification is how we become "more right on earth."

When we accept by faith God's simple plan of salvation, we are entitled to the benefits of sanctification. The primary benefit of justification is freedom from the *penalty of sin* but the primary benefit of sanctification is freedom from the *power of sin*. The benefits that come from submitting to God's process of sanctification are what lead us to the abundant life that Jesus promised to those who would live their life IN Christ Jesus.

To best explain how sanctification grants us His Power over sin and thus neutralizes the need to overcome sinful addictions in our own power, we will look at the **same six key words** that we defined in our last chapter. Each of these words that we defined in justification will be used to define both sanctification and glorification, as well.

SIN

Do Christians commit sin? The Bible tells us that after we are justified, we are now "made right in heaven". But, that does not make us automatically able to live right on earth. It is not by my power or might that I can avoid sinning, but by His Spirit that I can remain free from the power of sin. (See Zechariah 4:6.)

But, as believers, the issue is no longer whether or not we *commit* sin, but rather whether or not we willingly *permit* sin. (See First John 3:9.) Let me explain what that means. God has given every believer access to His Spirit of Power over the dormant power of sin that remains in our bodies. This wonder-working Power is harnessed within my inner man in the form of God's Holy Spirit. Wrong desires from outside pressure (temptations and trials) after my conversion continue to stimulate my mind to think wrong thoughts. But, it is when my mind chooses to *submit* to that stimulation that I have made the choice to *permit* sin. (See Romans 7:15-17.)

In others words, before we ever *do* wrong, we FIRST choose to *think* wrong! Thus, we do wrong before we actually *did* wrong, if you know what I mean. So, you can see that as Christians, it is not so much that we are sin *committers*. It is that we are choosing first to be sin *permitters*!

The Bible clearly teaches us that if we will not *permit* sin to enter into our thought processes, we will not *commit* those sins. Thus, the Power of God's Spirit is necessary to keep those thoughts from becoming constant daily meditations. (See Proverbs 23:7a.) If we think them, we will enter into unnecessary temptations that, if not handled properly, will lead us back to our addictive, sinful habits.

DEATH

Thinking wrong is a weakness of both the saved and the lost. But, it is the saved who have been given a guaranteed way of escape WITH the bad thoughts. (See First Corinthians 10:13.) Whenever outside pressure (oppression) stimulates our mind to think wrong, a discipled and developed Internal Presence from God will influence us to reject that outside pressure to sin. This "way of escape" will be provided WITH the temptation. Thus, at the same time we are tempted to think wrong, there is an exit ramp in our mind to get off the "road to eventual ruin." If we reject His "way of escape," we will pass by it and be forced to deal with the temptation in our own power. That is to say, we will have to find our own way of escape. Only our strong character can help us at this stage. And, if our will power is weak, we will probably soon commit that sin in our body, for we have permitted that sin to dwell in our mind. (See James 1:14-15)

In order to take the "way of escape" that the Power of His Presence provides, we must be willing to experience a death to self at the moment of His prompting in order to exit this road of ruin. We must literally be willing to **die to self** every day, and throughout the day. To die to self means to reject our selfish desires to think wrong.

So, we see that even as Christ died for us, we must also now be willing to **die *with* Christ**. (See Romans 6:6)

At Reformers Unanimous, our discipleship curriculum will teach you how you may experience that daily death that is a prerequisite for obtaining what the Bible calls the "Power of His resurrection." His Power can work through the life of a flawed man, but His Power works best through the life of a dead man! That is to say, a man that dies to his own selfishness.

When we die to self out of an unselfish desire to obey His promptings, we will experience a satisfaction of sorts. For we learn that when we suffer loss that we enjoy closer fellowship with Him. (See Philippians 3:8 and 10.) This period of intimate "fellowship of His suffering" represents our time of burial. Metaphorically, as we wait for God to empower us to get through a difficult situation, we are in a dormant position. We are dead to our own wishes but not yet alive in His Power. At this time, we are metaphorically secluded from the outside world and its ways, but we have a work going on with Christ in the darkness of our inner man.

This process, which I call our "time in the tomb" precedes the power that comes from His resurrected Life living through us. You may not understand this right now or quite see the symbolism of what I am teaching you, but as you grow and mature IN Christ through our addictions program, these truths will become real and personal to you.

So, we see that the Bible tells us that we are not only crucified *with* Christ as we die to self, but that we are also buried *with* Christ as He destroys the influences that want to control us. (See Romans 6:4) This time of waiting for His power is designed to be a sweet time of rest. But, for many believers, it is rejected and becomes, instead, a time of turbulent wrest.

At Reformers Unanimous, we will teach you through our discipleship curriculum how to patiently wait in your proverbial tomb as that which is "on your mind" may be starved of thought and eventually dissolve from your heart's meditation. When that wrong thought is no longer actively at work in your meditation, the enemy can no longer use it as a tool of manipulation. This allows you to experience the transformation process that grants you the Christ life that comes from His resurrection.

RESURRECTION

Sometimes we circumvent the resurrection process of the Christ Life when we choose to wrest *with* Christ rather than rest *in* Christ. We wrestle *with* Christ when, after we willingly die to self, but because of a difficult circumstance, we impatiently reject our time of waiting in the tomb for His power to come upon us. We, thus, yield to our own devices in order to overcome life's troubles. (See Proverbs 14:12)

We have died WITH Christ. We are buried WITH Christ and He intends for us to patiently await His timetable in order for us to be risen WITH Christ. (See Romans 6:4-5)

At Reformers Unanimous, we will teach you through our training and discipleship curriculum how to patiently wait on the Lord to renew your strength. This process of waiting on Him will surely give us the power that RU promises is available to us to overcome our stubborn habits and addictions. This is a truth you must believe if you are going to see any lasting change take place IN you.

BELIEVE

It takes belief, that is to say, faith, to save us. But, it also takes faith to change us. Before we are saved, we have very little faith. After we are saved, we are given the "faith of Christ" as one of the nine Fruit of the Holy Spirit. (See Galatians 5:22)

The term "Hidden life" is the daily death from our own affections and lusts in order to experience the Spirit Life. The Spirit Life comes from patiently resting in state for His Power to perform a good work in us. It is when we are "Hid-IN-Life."

To engage in this Hidden Life, we must exercise more dependence on Him than what it took to save us. But, this is not an increased dependence that is "quantitive". For dependence is dependence. But, rather, it is an increased dependence that is "durative". The duration (or length) of our faith is longer and longer between our "bouts with doubt." This increase of duration in our trust IN Him takes place as we spiritually develop. But, it is not *our* faith in which we are learning to remain confident. It is *His* faith that I must submit myself unto in order to experience the benefits of my sanctification. It takes my faith IN Christ to save me, but it takes *the* faith OF Christ to change me. (See Galatians 2:20 and Philippians 3:9.)

At Reformers Unanimous, our goal is to develop you out of your unbelief. There are many things that our human minds do not immediately comprehend. But, His faith that dwells within our spirit must operate independent of our feelings which dwell within our soul. When we know that God says something is true, we must accept it with the faith that He has placed within us. We cannot do this without a relationship IN Him.

At RU, our discipleship curriculum will help you develop that intimate and abiding love relationship with Jesus Christ. If you will believe *in* Him, you receive *from* Him.

RECEIVE

Jesus said that He came that we might have life, and that we might have it more abundantly. (See John 10:10) When we refuse to die *with* Christ, or to lie *with* Christ, or to rise *with* Christ, then our Christian life will be up and down, at best. That is not the *abundant* life; that is the *redundant* life. I want to receive what God has given unto me—eternal life. That life begins at conversion. But, in order to enjoy eternal life before I get to heaven, I must be willing to *do* as Christ *did*. Die, be buried, and be raised to walk in newness of life. (See Romans 6:4) If I yield to His faith in me, then I will receive His life living through me.

When we receive Christ as our Savior, the Holy Spirit will begin to persuade us through intuition, conviction, and worship. Whenever we reject any aspect of our selfless death, patient burial, and empowered resurrection, we stunt that internal persuasion and hinder our ability to live holy (soberly, righteously, and godly) in this present world. (See Titus 2:12) This will not separate us from God's presence, but it will strain His persuasion over us. We remain sanctified (set apart), but we no longer enjoy the benefits of our sanctification—abundant life, free from the power of sin and addiction.

At Reformers Unanimous, we *do not* help **addicts** live free from sin and addiction. We help **Christians** free live from sin and addiction. If you are a Christian, we believe this program can be a great help to you.
However, for RU to be of service to anyone, one must be willing to continue in this lifelong process of changing the way that we think. At RU, our goal is to help us overcome our "stinkin' thinking" by teaching everyone the biblical way to "tinker with your thinker."

At RU, we want to walk *with* you in our pilgrimage through sanctification. Together we will spiritually develop so that we may overcome all our crippling and habitual sins. Doing so brings us to our final chapter and benefit of salvation—glorification.

With our justification, we have BEEN saved from the PENALTY of sin. With our sanctification, we are BEING saved from the POWER of sin. Our third benefit is the future benefit of glorification. In glorification we shall BE saved from the PRESENCE of sin.

THE TRUTH
OUR REFORMATION THROUGH GLORIFICATION

This final benefit of glorification is the potential to glorify God in this life and the privilege to be glorified by God in the life hereafter. Our chapter title explains that we will be "reformed' thru glorification. Reformed is a key word at Reformers Unanimous, for it makes up the first word in our program's name.

Webster's dictionary defines the word *reform* to mean "to change from worse to better; to bring from a bad to a good state; to improve corrupt manners or morals, to remove that which is bad or corrupt; as, to reform abuses and to reform from vices."

That is a long definition that teaches us what God intends to do in our life. At RU, we hope to assist you in that process whereby God will "change you in more ways than just one." RU does not only focus on developing you from a drug addict to a sober living citizen, though we will focus on your recovery.

At RU, we want to help you experience much more change than that! We want to see you go from being unsaved to saved. We want you to go from headed to Hell to being Heaven-bound! We want you to go from being a self-focused person to a person focused on others. Yes, and we want you to go from being a bad person to a good person.

This is a process whereby we focus on our spiritual development as well as our personal development. The process of spiritual development has been explained in the previous two chapters of this book. It will also be taught more thoroughly as you engage in our Strongholds Discipleship Program curriculum. In this chapter however, we want to discuss the level of personal development that should follow your Strongholds Course work. The graduate's course work at RU is entitled, "Gaining Remaining Fruit." It is a focus on developing any missing character qualities you may not have in your life. Character qualities are necessary building blocks that God intends for us to learn as children. But, for some people, they fail to have them taught or they have rejected them till much later in life. We want to help you "reform" your character, where needed, from bad to good.

The second word in our program name is "unanimous." The word *unanimous* means "being of one mind." What that means is that at RU we are all unanimously focused on one thing—change! But, it is not a change that is acquired in our own effort, but it is a change that is granted to us by God, through His Spirit for Jesus' sake. We all strive for the mind of Christ. It is this mind that should be within us all. (See Philippians 2:5)

This change requires only one thing from us—a two-fold belief. A confession that believes *on* Jesus through His blood for our justification to save us and a conviction to believe *in* Jesus through His Spirit for our sanctification to change us. When we accept these commitments and believe with all our heart, lasting change is the natural result. That is when the glorification of God begins.

The word *glory* means to "bring the right opinion of." It literally means to "make God look good." The day will come when we will be saved not only from the penalty of sin (our justification), not only from the power of sin (our sanctification), but also from the presence of sin (our glorification). Until the day we enter Heaven's gate, our focus should not be on OUR glorification but rather on HIS glorification!

The Bible tells us that everything God created was intended to bring Him glory, to make Him look good. That is not the goal of many people's lives today, but God wants that to be our goal. We should strive to meet that goal by trusting in Him to reform us into God-glorifying new creatures in Christ.

With that said, sanctification is the key to glorification. If you are developing a dynamic love relationship with Jesus Christ, you will glorify God in your life. However, there will be times when your walk is weak or the adversity is particularly strong. We like to say at RU that "new levels bring new devils." At times like this, if we don't have strong character to lean on in spiritually weak times, we will be tempted to do things that may eventually lead us back to our addictive behavior. We may not "use" right away, but if we are not quick to make it right with God, we may grow farther from Him and engage in our sins of choice shortly thereafter.

During this process, which is called spiritual backsliding, we will need to have developed some character if we are going to remain *doing* right as we strive to *get* right. Now, please be advised that strong character is no substitute for strong Christianity. But, without strong character, we will be powerless when God's power is not granted to us.

Most addicts have character in some areas, but lack character in other areas. For example, you may have strong character traits like punctuality, initiative, good work ethic, or attentiveness. But, you may struggle in other areas like rebellion to authority, selfishness, pride, laziness, or jealousy. You can't glorify God especially during difficult times in your life if your weak character fails to improve. Your frustrations will overwhelm you and you will not do right unless circumstances change.

God may not want your circumstances to change. In Christ, you don't have to do right, you just have to submit to desiring to do right, and then He does the work for you. However, if we are not abiding IN Christ, we are not right with God. It takes character to *do* right when you are not right. At times like this, you are the one doing right. This is not God's choice, but it is better than doing wrong. It won't produce joy, but it will keep you from the consequences of sins done in the body. So, character development is important, especially for those who have very little.

However, the Bible says the Spirit of God WILL "sustain your infirmities." That word **infirmities** means "weaknesses." Our indwelling Spirit is strong enough to help us overcome our character weaknesses, even though we may remain personally insufficient to do so in our own power. At RU, we want you to learn to overcome those personal weaknesses as well as spiritually develop. It is designed for your own personal development.

This effort is made on your part by engaging in our graduate's course curriculum. We have two courses for our students. The entry level course is entitled "Strongholds," which is focused on developing the "fruits of the Spirit," which produces "righteousness." But, the graduate's course is entitled, "Gaining Remaining Fruit," which is focused on developing the "fruits of righteousness," which is godly Christian character. This course is designed to help you determine which missing character qualities might drift you back into your addiction during particularly difficult times in your spiritual pilgrimage.

Again, it is important that you understand that any character qualities we may fail to develop as young people are now of secondary importance to being a good Christian. Many people have good character but they may not be good Christians. We only glorify God when people see the strength of our Spirit, not the strength of our soul. In other words, we cannot exhibit the glorification of God to others without first enjoying the benefits of the sanctification of His Spirit—that is to say the benefits that come from developing an intimate personal relationship with Christ. Those benefits are the fruit (which means, "outcome or result") of the Spirit: love, joy, peace, longsuffering, gentleness, goodness, faith, meekness, and temperance.

So, we see that in order for our life to bring God glory right now, we must first focus on developing ourselves spiritually. Now at the same time, God will work on developing our personal lives to become stronger. This combination will be the best way to *stay* strong lest you *stray* weak!

At RU, we look forward to the opportunity of assisting you to spiritually develop first and foremost, and to personally develop you thereafter. However, someday there will be an even better experience for you my friend; and that is eternal glorification!

Someday all believers will glorify God in EVERYTHING that we do FOREVERMORE! The word *glorification* means almost the same thing as glory, or glorify. It means "to exalt one in honor and esteem." Someday, all believers will be exalted to a position where we will ALWAYS bring God honor and esteem. That day will come upon our physical death or His eminent return to earth in what the Bible calls "the rapture." Your RU leadership can explain what that means to you. It will be the most exciting time of your life, I can promise you that.

To date, all but two people who have gone into Heaven have done so as a result of their own physical death. In other words, they have died and awoken in Heaven, so to speak. When a believer's physical life ends, their body dies and their soul enters into Heaven's abode where they will forever bring Him glory.

When we accept God's simple plan of salvation, He does give us the power we need to glorify Him with our lives. It is even God's purpose for leaving us here for so long after our conversions—that others might see Him IN us and believe on His name. This brings God great glory here on earth.

But, from time to time, our lack of faith during particularly difficult times will lead us into failure in certain areas of our lives. At times like this, we will fail to glorify God. Likewise, we will be a disappointment to ourselves.

You see, the Power we need to glorify God comes from being completely yielded to Him. Remaining completely and unequivocally yielded to God is impossible when sin's presence is still alive in our bodies and actively trying to influence our lives.

However, when we are "lifted up to heaven," we will FINALLY experience freedom from the *presence of sin*. This future benefit grants us the sinless perfection that God originally designed for each of us to enjoy. In order to explain how to glorify God here on earth and how the glorification of God in Heaven actually works, allow me to use the same key words that we explained in our chapters on *Transformation through Justification* and *Conformation through Sanctification*.

SIN

When we are glorifying God, it is because sin has no dominion over us at a particular time. Its power has been rendered useless for we have chosen to die to the selfish desires of our soul and to yield to the depth of the personal relationship we have established in Christ through faith.

This means that the grace of God has taken over our life and is giving us the power to cast down the imaginations that usually stimulate us to yield to a particular temptation. This is not a once-for-all experience. When we allow our faith to waver to a form of doubt or blatant unbelief in Him, then our relationship suffers and adversity will be much harder to overcome.

Our improved character may keep us from outwardly sinning or even quickly sinning. But, eventually, if we do no rectify the mistakes we are making in our walk with God, then our character will grow weak. This will leave us vulnerable to the internal sin of wrong thinking. Once again, this wrong thinking is found in the meditations of our heart.

Shortly after our wrong meditations begin we will probably give into this contemplation of temptation. When this happens, we will not glorify God for we are no longer under His power. Thus we cannot maintain a righteous lifestyle. It is impossible to live godly in our own power.

This compromise leads us to *permit* sinful thoughts in our mind to overcome the meditations of our heart. Once we permit ourselves to think about sin with any lengthy duration whatsoever, it will eventually cause us to *commit* that sin in our body. It was earlier explained that, when we permit sin to control our heart, we are already engaging in wrong behavior. Thus we will soon commit that wrong. But, we have already permitted ourselves to *being* wrong before we commit ourselves to *doing* wrong. To "be holy" we must give our minds over to God. To "be unholy" we must give our minds over to the things of this world.

This internal permitting of sin in our mind is what separates us from fellowship with God and hinders the Spirit's ability to glorify God with our life. That is how sin will stunt our ability to glorify God here on earth.

However, when Christ shall come, all believers shall see a change take place "in the air." That change will eradicate our sin nature. This means that when we enter heaven, we will have been forever saved from the *presence* of sin. Once again, this rapture really should be explained to you by your RU leader.

DEATH

There are two types of death that lead to glorification. One type of death glorifies God and the other will bring us glorification. Let's first look at the death that brings glory to God. We have discussed it earlier, as well. It is the death of self. When we commit ourselves to dying to oneself and choose rather to live by the prompting of our indwelling Holy Spirit, we are experiencing the benefits of conforming through our sanctification. Some believers do that often, others sometimes, and some hardly ever. Those who rarely die to self do not bring glory to God. Even when they are able to do right, those who know them best recognize it as a seldom experienced victory and will be skeptical of their good works. This will not glorify God. They know the person well enough to know they cannot maintain the consistency that comes only from dying daily to our own selfish wants.

So, God may receive a small measure of glory, but it soon fades as that person falls back into their fleshly, stubborn ways. This is not the type of occasional dying experience that God wants from us. He wants us to die to self every day, throughout the day.

But, we are unable to do so unless we develop a deep abiding relationship with Jesus Christ that manifests itself in wanting what He wants, thinking like He thinks, and feeling the way He feels. We need to nurture our nature to be more like Christ, not by changing our life but by exchanging our life for His life!

The Bible says that when we are crucified spiritually we are crucified WITH Christ. Though we are still alive physically, it is Him that has come to life spiritually. Thus, it is Christ that is supposed to be living His life within me. The Bible says that Christ living in me is the hope of glory. The word *hope* means "expectation." The only expectation I have for bringing God glory is for Christ to live IN me that I may submit to allowing Him to live FOR me. That is the "hid-in-life" we teach at RU.

To bring God glory, not once for a little while, but regularly for long periods, we need to die to self, as prompted by God. This takes a commitment to following the Spirit's leading while learning how to "walk after the Spirit." This is how we glorify God with our lives. It is the Christ Life being accessed through our own personal death to the self life.

However, if we physically perish before Christ returns, then upon our death, it is our human body that experiences death. If we are believers, as outlined in our chapter on transformation thru justification, our soul will never die. Our soul has been spared its much deserved death as a result of our accepting Christ payment on the cross. (See James 5:20.)

Though our body parts will cease to function and we will be buried as we experience our physical death, the soul is incorruptible, it never dies. Our soul will take on immortality in a perfect state as promised by God in His Word. (See First Corinthians 15:53.)

This death will bring US glorification, which once again, is freedom from the presence of sin. However, after our spiritual daily death or our physical once-in-a-lifetime death, there will be a time of burial.

BURIAL

When we die to our selfish wants and wishes, we will be at a proverbial crossroads. At this stage we can climb off that cross as a dead man and resurrect our lives in our power and begin "trying hard to do better." But, if we do this, we will only fail again and again with no real sign of victory. Or, we can patiently wait for God's power to come upon us before we advance down the right path at that crossroads. The timing of our outside pressure to *do* wrong and our internal persuasion to *be* right comes simultaneously.

But, as a result of a weakened walk, the internal persuasion is easily overlooked.

This ought not to be. The Bible says a wise man see evil coming and hides himself from it. But, naive people pass on and receive a punishment for the error of their ways. If we are going to glorify God with our lives, we must be willing to die and remain buried until Christ resurrects Himself in us. The Apostle Paul (one of the men that God used to pen the words of the Bible) said he died daily, but he never said he resurrected daily. For it was not him that resurrected but rather it was Him!

RESURRECTION

Though we may wrestle with Christ in our own power and have a tendency during times of weak faith to falter as a result, God is faithful to not suffer us to be tempted with more than we can handle. As a result, our stubbornness when being unselfish will bring us great conviction or even adversity that is clearly the chastening of the Lord. At this time, we are more willing to "get it over with" and die spiritually that we may resurrect with Him. If we take this process through its supernatural course, then we will patently wait for His indwelling Spirit to lead us out of our mistakes. This is our spiritual resurrection. It is our stubborn soul dying, and our developing spirit resurrecting and taking its rightful role of authority over our thoughts, wishes, and wants.

This process brings God *great* glory for at times like this we are humbling ourselves! Bold humility (Boldness is faith, and humility is trust in God rather than oneself) is the key to gaining grace and mercy in our times of need. (See Hebrews 4:16)

This humbling process will keep us from returning so quickly to the self reliance that brings us back to a position of pride. Returning back to our position of pride is what brings us to another painful crucifixion. Though a crucifixion for our wrong wishes brings God glory, nothing glorifies Him more than when our submission to His Spirit reveals to others a desire to abide deeper IN Him.

When we die or Christ returns, we will forever be glorified and free from the presence of sin. God's creation will once again function as He had created it in the beginning. Until that glorious day, we ought always to glorify God and not our own selves. This can only be done as we reject sin's *pressure* in our life and yield to God's *power* over sin's presence. This takes only submission to what we have chosen to believe during difficult circumstances.

BELIEVE

My friend, have you believed that Jesus Christ can transform your life thorough the salvation experience of justification? If so, you are born again and you have BEEN saved from the PENALTY of sin, which is death and Hell.

If you have been saved through the faith found in justification, have you also chosen to begin a relationship with Him in which you are learning to follow His leading? If you are doing so, or are committed to do so, then my friend, you are BEING saved from the POWER of sin.

And, finally, are you committed to having a long-term walk with God by yielding yourself to that developing relationship with God's Son through His Spirit? If you do this with regularity and reject compromise in your thought life, then my friend, you will bring God great glory in this life. You have been reformed by your desires to make Him look good with your life!

Your next and final benefit remains to be seen. It will be the day and time when you and I and Dr. Crabb and many untold others will be glorified. It is at that time we will BE saved from the PRESENCE of sin. Until that day, I ask of God that peace be with you. Not a temporary peace that any program may be able to grant you, but the "Peace that passes understanding". It comes only from God as we enjoy and experience all the benefits of your salvation.

The Transformation of Justification: Have you **been saved** from sin's *penalty*? If not, then you need to be justified. If you have been justified, then you will be **judged as a** child of God and saved from sin's *penalty*.

The Conformation of Sanctification: Are you also **being saved** from sin's *power*? If not, then you need to enjoy the primary benefit that comes from sanctification. It is a deep abiding personal relationship with Him that manifests itself in victory over vice. We will make mistakes and find ourselves being **judged as a son**. However, God will develop us like the loving Father He is to be the son we never thought we could be. This development will save us regularly from sin's *power*.

Our Reformation Through Glorifiacation | 232

The Reformation of Glorification: Are you victorious in life, enjoying the abundant Christian life? If so, then you are avoiding the disruption that can be caused by sin's presence in the members of your body. That is to be commended. However, the day will come when we will all be **judged as a servant**. How did we serve others? This will take place after our glorification when we **will be saved** from sin's *presence*.

I know that not all of these truths will be easily or even immediately understood by all who read this book. Very few will have even heard a great many of the facts found in this book, backed up by the Scriptures found in the back of the book. However, that doesn't matter. If you are willing and wanting to learn more about the Truth, He will be revealed to you at a pace that God feels is appropriate for you.

Right now, you may receive from God what the Bible refers to as the "milk of the Word." But, His Word teaches us that as we use it regularly, we will mature to what the Bible calls "strong meat." The truths taught in this book may start as milk and become quite meaty. Worry not. We at RU are here to help you on this journey. And, when your pilgrimage is over, you will be quite pleased with what God has done for you.

In conclusion, I surely hope you will study this book over and over again. And, if you visited one of our chapters recently, we hope to see you again next week.

Proverbs 14:12 *There is a way which seemeth right unto a man, but the end thereof are the ways of death.*

Proverbs 23:7a *For as he thinketh in his heart, so is he.*

Ezekiel 36:27 *And I will put my spirit within you, and cause you to walk in my statutes, and ye shall keep my judgments, and do them.*

Zechariah 4:6 *Then he answered and spake unto me, saying, This is the word of the LORD unto Zerubbabel, saying, Not by might, nor by power, but by my spirit, saith the LORD of hosts.*

Matthew 27:62 *Now the next day, that followed the day of the preparation, the chief priests and Pharisees came together unto Pilate,*

Matthew 27:63 *Saying, Sir, we remember that that deceiver said, while he was yet alive, After three days I will rise again.*

Matthew 27:64 *Command therefore that the sepulchre be made sure until the third day, lest his disciples come by night, and steal him away, and say unto the people, He is risen from the dead: so the last error shall be worse than the first.*

Matthew 27:65 *Pilate said unto them, Ye have a watch: go your way, make it as sure as ye can.*

Matthew 28:5 *And the angel answered and said unto the women, Fear not ye: for I know that ye seek Jesus, which was crucified.*
Matthew 28:6 *He is not here: for he is risen, as he said. Come, see the place where the Lord lay.*

Matthew 28:7 *And go quickly, and tell his disciples that he is risen from the dead; and, behold, he goeth before you into Galilee; there shall ye see him: lo, I have told you.*

John 3:16 *For God so loved the world, that he gave his only begotten Son, that whosoever believeth in him should not perish, but have everlasting life.*

John 8:32 *And ye shall know the truth, and the truth shall make you free.*

John 8:36 *If the Son therefore shall make you free, ye shall be free indeed.*

John 10:10 *The thief cometh not, but for to steal, and to kill, and to destroy: I am come that they might have life, and that they might have it more abundantly.*

John 14:16 *And I will pray the Father, and he shall give you another Comforter, that he may abide with you for ever;*

Romans 3:23 *For all have sinned, and come short of the glory of God;*

Romans 5:8 *But God commendeth his love toward us, in that, while we were yet sinners, Christ died for us.*

Romans 5:12 *Wherefore, as by one man sin entered into the world, and death by sin; and so death passed upon all men, for that all have sinned:*
Romans 6:4 *Therefore we are buried with him by baptism into death: that like as Christ was raised up from the dead by the glory of the Father, even so we also should walk in newness of life.*

Romans 6:5 *For if we have been planted together in the likeness of his death, we shall be also in the likeness of his resurrection:*

Romans 6:6 *Knowing this, that our old man is crucified with him, that the body of sin might be destroyed, that henceforth we should not serve sin.*

Romans 6:23 *For the wages of sin is death; but the gift of God is eternal life through Jesus Christ our Lord.*

Romans 7:15 *For that which I do I allow not: for what I would, that do I not; but what I hate, that do I.*

Romans 7:16 *If then I do that which I would not, I consent unto the law that it is good.*

Romans 7:17 *Now then it is no more I that do it, but sin that dwelleth in me.*

Romans 10:9 *That if thou shalt confess with thy mouth the Lord Jesus, and shalt believe in thine heart that God hath raised him from the dead, thou shalt be saved.*

Romans 12:2 *And be not conformed to this world: but be ye transformed by the renewing of your mind, that ye may prove what is that good, and acceptable, and perfect, will of God.*

1 Corinthians 10:13 *There hath no temptation taken you but such as is common to man: but God is faithful, who will not suffer you to be tempted above that ye are able; but will with the temptation also make a way to escape, that ye may be able to bear it.*

1 Corinthians 15:53 *For this corruptible must put on incorruption, and this* *mortal must put on immortality.*

Galatians 2:20 *I am crucified with Christ: nevertheless I live; yet not I, but Christ liveth in me: and the life which I now live in the flesh I live by the faith of the Son of God, who loved me, and gave himself for me.*

Galatians 5:22 *But the fruit of the Spirit is love, joy, peace, longsuffering, gentleness, goodness, faith.*

Philippians 3:8 *Yea doubtless, and I count all things but loss for the excellency of the knowledge of Christ Jesus my Lord: for whom I have suffered the loss of all things, and do count them but dung, that I may win Christ,*

Philippians 3:9 *And be found in him, not having mine own righteousness, which is of the law, but that which is through the faith of Christ, the righteousness which is of God by faith:*

Philippians 3:10 *That I may know him, and the power of his resurrection, and the fellowship of his sufferings, being made conformable unto his death;*

Titus 2:12 *Teaching us that, denying ungodliness and worldly lusts, we should live soberly, righteously, and godly, in this present world;*
Hebrews 4:16 *Let us therefore come boldly unto the throne of grace, that we may obtain mercy, and find grace to help in time of need.*

James 1:14 *But every man is tempted, when he is drawn away of his own lust, and enticed.*

James 1:15 *Then when lust hath conceived, it bringeth forth sin: and sin, when it is finished, bringeth forth death.*

James 5:20 *Let him know, that he which converteth the sinner from the error of his way shall save a soul from death, and shall hide a multitude of sins.*

1 Peter 3:18 *For Christ also hath once suffered for sins, the just for the unjust, that he might bring us to God, being put to death in the flesh, but quickened by the Spirit:*

1 John 3:9 *Whosoever is born of God doth not commit sin; for his seed remaineth in him: and he cannot sin, because he is born of God.*

1 John 5:1 *Whosoever believeth that Jesus is the Christ is born of God: and every one that loveth him that begat loveth him also that is begotten of him.*

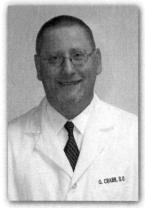

George Crabb D.O., F.A.C.O.I.
Addiction Medicine Specialist

Dr. George T. Crabb is a Board Certified Internal Medicine physician and a Fellow of the American College of Osteopathic Internist. He practices Internal Medicine and Addiction Medicine in Naples, Florida. He is a member of the American Society of Addiction Medicine, the American Osteopathic Academy of Addiction Medicine, and the Florida Osteopathic Medical Association.

Dr. Crabb serves as the Medical Advisor to Reformers Unanimous International Ministry. He has an active pulpit ministry and frequently speaks abroad representing the RUI Ministry. Dr. Crabb conducts seminars on a wide range of medical and spiritual topics. Many of his seminars are available on DVD through the RUI web site (www.reformersrecovery.com.) He has a website filled with helpful, Biblically based information regarding topics such as addiction, physical health and spiritual matters (www.drgeorgecrabb.com.) He has authored several books and numerous booklets all published through the RUI Ministry and available through their web site. He continues to write and edit medical communications for the RUI Ministry.

Dr. Crabb is an ordained Baptist minister. He served with his father (Pastor Dr. George Crabb, Antioch Baptist Church, Warren, MI) as an assistant for nearly 20 years prior to moving to Rockford, Illinois in 2008. While in Rockford he worked closely with Pastor Dr. Paul Kingsbury, Bro. Steve Curington and Bro. Ben Burks before God led him and his family to Naples, Florida in 2010. Dr. Crabb and his family are actively serving God through a local church in Naples. He has also received certification through the Drug Enforcement Agency (DEA) to detoxify individuals (done in the privacy of his office) who are addicted to any form of opiate based drugs using the medication called Suboxone (buprenorphine/naloxone – www.suboxone.com). Individuals, including many pastors and RU directors, leaders and students throughout the United States, Canada and the United Kingdom have sought out his counsel and medical treatment. He is currently practicing Internal Medicine and Addiction Medicine through the NCH Healthcare Group, Naples, Florida (www.nchmd.org).

Dr. Crabb's passion has always been to help others through the liberating truth of Jesus Christ. Jesus said, "I am come that they might have life, and that they might have it more abundantly." (John 10:10)

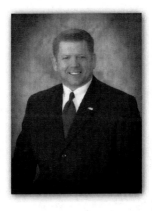

Steven Boyd Curington
RUI Founder
October 1, 1965-October 30, 2010

Steve grew up in Rockford, Illinois, and attended North Love Christian School. Upon graduation, Steve walked away from the truths he had learned and thus began a 10-year drug addiction. After a serious car accident, Steve was delivered from his addiction through the support of North Love Baptist Church and the truth found in John 8:32, *"And ye shall know the truth, and the truth shall make you free."*

Because of his newfound freedom, Steve was burdened to reach out to others. Thus, he began a small Bible study in his local church in 1996. This grew and developed and has now reached out to thousands within our local community who have struggled with stubborn habits and addiction.

In 2000, this Friday night program, complete with curriculum, began to be implemented into other communities across the country. Many were finding freedom from things that once held them bound. During the course of Steve's life, he initiated the starting of over 800 Reformers Unanimous local chapters that meet every Friday night across the globe.

With natural leadership and unflagging determination, Steve also saw the need for a residential treatment program in Rockford to restore broken lives. He secured what is affectionately known as Mulberry, an 18-bedroom apartment building. Then, he facilitated the purchase of a nursing home on Safford Road that houses up to 100 men. And just recently, Steve secured a second nursing home on Arnold Street to house up to 80 women. These three locations, once broken down and vacated, are now beautifully restored like the lives of those who live there and victoriously graduate the program.

The plight of the incarcerated could not be overlooked. Steve also developed what is known as the Reformers Institutional Program (RIP) curriculum that is used nationwide for the incarcerated to help stop the recidivism. Many have found freedom behind bars through his teaching and discipleship.

Since its inception, RUI has worked to improve the quality of life for communities worldwide by providing an array of services for those suffering from the effects of addictions. Each week, these "chapters" serve an average of 32,000 people who are affected by addictions, and incorporate the help of over 5,000 volunteers. These individual Friday night programs, as well as the residential programs, not only help the individual seeking help, but also the numerous friends and family members whose lives are affected by the addiction of their loved one. Families have been restored and relationships have been salvaged as a result of Reformers Unanimous.

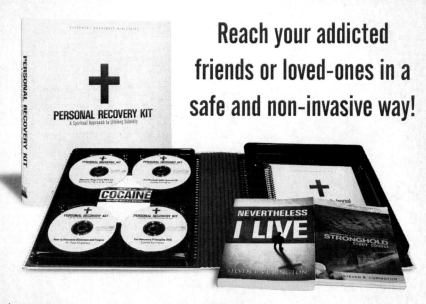

Reach your addicted friends or loved-ones in a safe and non-invasive way!

- ▶ Topical Addiction Recovery Book (15 topics from which to choose: from alcohol, cocaine, meth, marijuana, cutting, pornography, stimulants, tobacco, eating disorders, gambling, prescription meds, heroin, acid, huffing, and steroids)
- ▶ Spiritual Recovery Journal w/ instructional CD
- ▶ Spiritual Recovery Textbook
- ▶ 10 Spiritual Recovery Principles DVD
- ▶ Spiritual Recovery Program Workbook
- ▶ Bitterness and Forgiveness Recovery Series on MP3 CD
- ▶ Spiritual Recovery Mega-Pack on MP3 CD (Includes topical teaching on: wrong thinking, depression, forgiveness, Rx addiction, sexual addiction, opiates, and dozens of other topics.)

$99.⁰⁰

This proven method is a great way to introduce your loved-one to the life-saving ministry of Reformers Unanimous in a simple, non-invasive manner. Ask God if He would have you intervene in your loved one's life, and allow Reformers Unanimous to present the saving power of Jesus Christ in an easy and convenient way. Do not delay, my friends…lives rest in the balance!!!

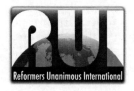

Reformers Unanimous International

call **815-986-0460**
or visit **www.personalrecoverykit.com**

DO YOU NEED TO GET AWAY FROM IT ALL?
HOW ABOUT FAR AWAY?

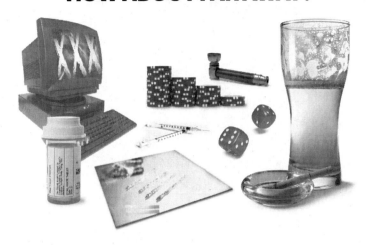

REFORMERS UNANIMOUS
Schools of Discipleship for Men and Women
A distinctively Bible-based program

If you or someone else needs the kind of
help that only a residential
program can provide, please contact our
offices at **815-986-0460.**
Don't hesitate... a life may depend on it.

**The Men's and Women's Discipleship Homes are
located in** *Rockford, Illinois*

to download an application visit ruhomes.org

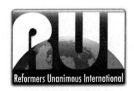

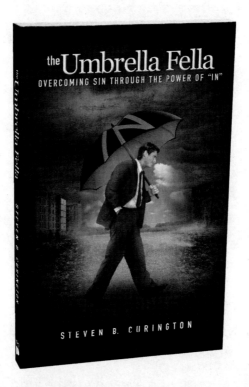

The Umbrella Fella (CE-123) $12.00

Within every believer's heart is a desire to be all that God would have us to be. But, how can we be what God wants us to be, when we cannot even do the things God wants us to do?! The Umbrella Fella will help us better understand our position in the kingdom of Heaven's chain of command. Once we understand our position, it will forever change our disposition. It all begins with a two letter preposition, the little word – IN.

15 Relevant Topical Books on Addiction

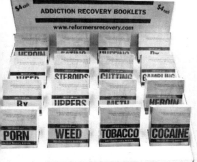

Renowned addiction experts Steven Curington and Dr. George Crabb D.O., break apart the effects that addiction plays on the body, the soul, and the spirit. By introducing the full gospel of justification, sanctification, and glorification to the recovering addict, an individual learns the effects that Jesus Christ can produce within our spirit, soul, and body.

This makes an ideal witnessing and recovery tool for lost addicts and their loved ones.

Topical Books – **$4.**⁰⁰ each
One Complete Set – **$45.**⁰⁰

Display Stand – **$20.**⁰⁰
3 of Each Book w/Display Stand – **$149.**⁰⁰

As a doctor, I'm always looking for an effective and non-invasive way of helping and witnessing to addicted patients and their loved ones. I have found a tool in these topical books that is both scripturally and medically sound. I would recommend them to any doctor looking to impart spiritual as well as physical well being.
– Dr. Morris Harper, Communicable Disease Specialist

Reformers Unanimous International

o order call **(815) 986-0460** or visit **reformersrecovery.com**

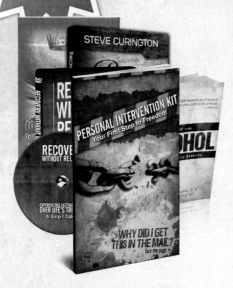